D1197554

Perfect Detox

Gill Paul is the author of several health and nutrition books. She has road-tested a wide selection of detox methods and theories.

Other titles in the *Perfect* series

Perfect Answers to Interview Questions – Max Eggert
Perfect Babies' Names – Rosalind Fergusson
Perfect Best Man – George Davidson
Perfect Brain Training – Philip Carter
Perfect Calorie Counting – Kate Santon
Perfect Confidence – Jan Ferguson
Perfect CV – Max Eggert
Perfect Family Quiz – David Pickering
Perfect Interview – Max Eggert
Perfect Letters and Emails for all Occasions – George Davidson
Perfect Memory Training – Fiona McPherson
Perfect Numerical and Logical Test Results – Joanna Moutafi and Marianna Moutafi
Perfect Numerical Test Results – Joanna Moutafi and Ian Newcombe
Perfect Party Games – Stephen Curtis
Perfect Personality Profiles – Helen Baron
Perfect Persuasion – Richard Storey
Perfect Positive Thinking – Lynn Williams
Perfect Presentations – Andrew Leigh and Michael Maynard
Perfect Psychometric Test Results – Joanna Moutafi and Ian Newcombe
Perfect Pub Quiz – David Pickering
Perfect Punctuation – Stephen Curtis
Perfect Readings for Weddings – Jonathan Law
Perfect Relaxation – Elaine van der Zeil
Perfect Speeches for All Occasions - Matt Shinn
Perfect Wedding Planning – Cherry Chappell
Perfect Wedding Speeches and Toasts – George Davidson
Perfect Weight Loss – Kate Santon
Perfect Written English – Chris West

Perfect
Detox

Gill Paul

BOOKS

Published by Random House Books 2009
1 2 3 4 5 6 7 8 9 10

Copyright © Grapevine Publishing Services 2009

Gill Paul has asserted her right under the Copyright, Designs and
Patents Act, 1988, to be identified as the author of this work

This book is sold subject to the condition that it shall not, by way of
trade or otherwise, be lent, resold, hired out, or otherwise circulated
without the publisher's prior consent in any form of binding or cover
other than that in which it is published and without a similar condition,
including this condition, being imposed on the subsequent purchaser.

First published in Great Britain in 2009 by
Random House Books
Random House, 20 Vauxhall Bridge Road,
London SW1V 2SA

www.rbooks.co.uk

Addresses for companies within The Random House Group Limited
can be found at: www.randomhouse.co.uk/offices.htm

The Random House Group Limited Reg. No. 954009

A CIP catalogue record for this book
is available from the British Library

ISBN 9781847945488

The Random House Group Limited makes every effort to ensure that
the papers used in its books are made from trees that have been legally
sourced from well-managed and credibly certified forests. Our paper
procurement policy can be found at
www.randomhouse.co.uk/paper.htm

Typeset by Delineate for Grapevine Publishing Services Ltd

Printed and bound in Great Britain by
CPI Bookmarque, Croydon, CR0 4TD

Contents

Introduction   6

1 How does detoxing work?   8
2 Your detox plan   28
3 Food and drink   47
4 Detox aids   57
Detox superfoods A–Z   82
Recipes   123
   Breakfast   124
   Lunch   127
   Dinner   132
   Salads   141
   Easy dressings, dips and sauces   145
   Puddings   153
   Fresh fruit and vegetable juices   156

Conclusion   158
Index   159

Introduction

Do you lack the energy you once had? Are you suffering from headaches, fatigue, niggling health problems, unexplained aches and pains, poor digestion, constipation or skin problems? Are you conscious that your diet isn't quite as good as it should be, and that you've hit the junk food, the bottle or a packet of cigarettes more often than you ought to? Do you seem to have put on weight squarely around your middle?

Perhaps you've been on long-term medication or a course of antibiotics; perhaps you are aware that you overuse chemicals – for cleaning your home, personal hygiene and even washing your clothes. Do you spend a lot of time breathing in fumes from traffic? Do you regularly have your clothing dry-cleaned? Or do you live in a highly polluted area? Do E-numbers form the basis of many of the foods you eat? Is water low on your list of favourite regular drinks? Are you aware that you don't drink enough water, full stop?

All and any of these are compelling reasons why *Perfect Detox* is right for you. We are surrounded by toxins in daily life and it's not surprising that they begin to have an impact on our overall health, affecting the organs in our bodies such as the liver, lungs, digestive system, skin and kidneys, that are designed to eliminate them. When our systems become compromised, toxins begin to build up and our bodies struggle to maintain balance. The result? Health problems, lack of energy, weight issues and a sluggish, stagnant system that affects our well-being on every level.

Perfect Detox is designed to spring-clean your body, giving it the nutrients it needs to perform at optimum level, removing toxins that have been stored, kick-starting, supporting and cleansing the organs that are responsible for elimination and getting things moving so that every system is working efficiently.

And what can you expect as a result? Niggling health problems will vanish, and you'll experience renewed energy and vigour; your skin will glow with good health and your body will begin to work effectively. If you are overweight, you can expect to lose some unwanted pounds, particularly around the middle of your body, where they tend to be stored when your liver is under pressure and you have been burning the candle at both ends. Best of all, you'll clear out debris, and that will leave your body feeling fresh and vital.

Whether you want a quick fix to undo some short-term damage, or something longer term to deep-clean a sluggish system and get it working the way it should, *Perfect Detox* is for you. We've got several plans to get the toxins moving and your body functioning well, with delicious recipes and suggestions for foods, supplements and other aids that will make the process that much easier. *Perfect Detox* doesn't require a massive lifestyle change; instead, you'll need to make some simple alterations to your diet, cutting out some of the nasties, and replacing them with nutritious, health-enhancing foods that will increase your vitality on every level. You'll get a taste of healthier new habits that will have an instant effect on the way you look and feel, and which you may wish to carry on with long after your perfect detox has finished. And that's where our handy maintenance tips come in. We'll help you to establish a programme that will enhance rather than detract from your health, and clear out the toxins long before they become a problem.

Now, let's get started!

1 How does detoxing work?

Our bodies are miraculous things, designed to heal themselves, fend off invaders such as viruses and bacteria, and to regenerate and renew. They are also designed to cope with a certain number of toxins – those naturally occurring in our foods and our environment, for example – by neutralising, transforming or eliminating them from the body. Our livers help to convert toxic substances into harmless ones, our intestines break down protein, carbohydrates and fats, while our kidneys filter waste from the bloodstream. We also eliminate toxins through our skin when we sweat and our lymphatic system clears debris from our blood. The immune system is involved in fighting off bacteria and other invaders.

A toxin is anything that obstructs or delays the normal functions of our bodies, or causes stagnation, congestion or disease. For example, we take in chemicals such as pesticides, household cleaners, food additives, drugs, pollution, cigarette smoke and heavy metals such as lead by breathing them, eating them or simply absorbing them through the skin. If we overload the systems that are designed to deal with toxins by making them work too hard, they accumulate in the body – and that's when problems start.

Toxic overload

In the modern world, toxicity or 'toxic overload' is a greater problem than it is has ever been before. Every day we are surrounded by a multitude of chemicals, many of which are strong and some of which are literally toxic, meaning poisonous or capable of causing damage to our bodies. We are exposed to air and water pollution, radiation (in the form of microwaves, radio waves and ultraviolet rays from the sun, for example) and nuclear power. Our diets are full of chemicals to keep food fresh, and to provide texture, consistency and flavour. We eat more sugar and refined foods, and rely on stimulants, such as coffee, tea and cola, as well as on sedatives such as alcohol to keep us going. What's more, when we become ill, we pop a painkiller or antibiotic that creates even more work for our bodies. We breathe chemicals, eat them and touch them every single day of our lives, no matter how careful we are about diet and lifestyle.

And there is more! Our bodies actually produce their own toxins as they go about the business of staying alive and these need to be eliminated. Bacteria, yeast and parasites produce waste that our bodies have to handle. Then there are substances called free radicals that must be expelled from the body. These atoms or groups of atoms cause damage to cells, impairing the immune system and leading to degenerative disorders such as heart disease and cancer. Free-radical damage is believed to accelerate the ageing process as well. There are a number of free radicals that are known to occur in the body. They may be formed by exposure to radiation and toxic chemicals, such as those found in cigarette smoke, overexposure to the sun's rays or various metabolic processes, such as the process of breaking down stored fat molecules for use as an energy source.

Toxic overload occurs when we have taken in more toxins than we can get rid of. Uneliminated toxins are stored in our tissues, and they can harm our overall health on a daily basis and sow the seeds of future illness. As more and more demands are placed on the body, an increasing amount of energy is required to deal with them. This is the same energy required for other body functions, such as breathing, digestion, excretion, cell growth and renewal, fighting off infection, thinking and moving. These processes are necessary for life, and our bodies are simply not designed to cope with the extra modern-day stresses placed upon them. Toxins build up, and body systems work ineffectively. This is one of the most common causes of low-grade niggling disease on a daily basis (insomnia, fatigue, irritability, headaches, digestive disorders, skin problems, poor concentration and susceptibility to common ailments, for example) and in the long term it can be responsible for broad-scale immune system failure and a host of debilitating diseases.

The role of the liver

Although there are many body systems responsible for removing toxins from the body, the liver is undoubtedly the most important, and the most hard-working. Weighing in at about 900g and situated behind the lower ribs on the right side, the liver is capable of regenerating its own tissue faster than any other organ of the body. It can also function with only 20 per cent of its original mass before we begin to notice any specific health problems.

It has a number of functions that are vital to life – some 500 in total – including aiding digestion and absorption of nutrients; storing essential vitamins and minerals; creating bile, which breaks down fats and excretes waste; helping to maintain electrolyte and water balance in the body; creating red blood cells and cleansing the blood; regulating cholesterol; processing and metabolising hormones as well as removing old hormones that are no longer needed; regulating blood sugar and working as part of the immune system to fight infection. The liver neutralises harmful substances in a complicated series of chemical reactions – it is crucial to the detoxification process.

The liver makes fat-soluble toxins into water-soluble ones, which means that they can be excreted from the body in urine or sweat. Fat-soluble toxins are stored in cell membranes and in body fat, sometimes for years, before being released when we exercise, are stressed or lose weight and start calling up fat stores for energy. The liver also filters the blood, removing invaders such as bacteria, fungi, viruses and parasites, and neutralises a wide range of toxic chemicals – from our food and drink, our environment and those produced by our bodies.

It's worth understanding how the liver detoxifies many harmful substances into less harmful forms which the body can safely eliminate.

There are two parts to this detoxification process: in phase I, enzymes activate toxic substances, making them more accessible to the next phase. Phase II continues this procedure, converting toxins to more water-soluble forms for elimination through urine and stools. There are a number of foods and herbs that can encourage this process, both phases of which must take place in order for toxins to be removed from our bodies.

It makes sense that our livers should be healthy and strong to do their job on a day-to-day basis, and that is one reason why a detox is important. Not only will you be encouraging your body to work more efficiently, but you will also be supporting and actually cleansing your liver. Need more encouragement? It is now believed that up to 90 per cent of all cancers are caused by the effects of environmental carcinogens – such as those found in cigarette smoke, water, food and air – in combination with a shortfall in the nutrients that our bodies need for our immune and detoxification systems to work effectively. It follows that proper functioning of the liver – our key detoxifying organ – could help prevent cancer.

Symptoms of an overworked or toxic liver

As our livers become overloaded, they become 'fatty' and calcified in places, meaning that they are unable to undertake their normal functions, of which detoxification is key. So toxins build up in our bodies, are stored in fat cells, and are then carried to vital organs through the bloodstream. As impurities enter the bloodstream, headaches and sluggishness are common. Because digestion is impaired, constipation occurs, which then allows toxins to re-enter the bloodstream from the intestines. From here, they affect every organ and system in the body, compromising the function of the brain, nervous and digestive systems, skin, immunity, circulation, energy levels, hormonal balance, fertility, metabolism and kidney function; bowel habits and blood sugar are also affected.

Another way that the liver can eliminate harmful substances is by excreting them into the bile. The gall bladder is a pear-shaped pouch for bile received from the liver, which, when secreted into the small intestines, helps to digest and break down fat and cholesterol. Bile salts contain cholesterol in a liquid form. However, if there is an excess of cholesterol and other toxins they can crystallise in the gall bladder. When this happens gallstones begin to form.

As the liver struggles to deal with toxins, we may become more sensitive to environmental toxins, experiencing allergies and allergic responses, feelings of lethargy and a lack of energy. And because the liver partly controls blood-sugar levels, in its overworked state it may struggle to maintain a constant level, leading to fluctuations that can affect energy levels enormously.

What's more, because digestion is less effective, our bodies will struggle to get the nutrients they need, which can lead to fatigue and illness. You may find that you wake up in the night to urinate because your overworked liver understimulates your kidneys, which causes them to become congested as well. Women may experience heavier periods, with clotting and cramps.

The common signs of an overworked liver include:

- Digestion and elimination problems including constipation, bloating, frequent urination, diarrhoea and nausea.
- Acid reflux and heartburn.
- Headaches.
- High cholesterol.
- Food cravings.
- Weight gain, particularly around the abdomen.
- Cellulite.
- Eye problems, including spots, floaters, dry eyes, cataracts and sore eyes.
- Blood-sugar imbalances.
- Hormonal imbalances, which can manifest themselves as PMS, fertility problems, extreme menopause symptoms (hot flushes, night sweats) and heavy periods.
- Allergies, such as hay fever, hives, skin rashes and asthma.
- Fluid retention.

- Skin disorders, including rashes, spider veins, darkened patches of skin known as 'liver spots', dryness.
- Repeated infections.
- Muscle and/or joint pain.
- Bad breath and body odour.
- Dark circles under the eyes.
- Chemical sensitivities.
- Depression, anger and irritability – the result of toxins reaching the brain, hormonal imbalance and blood-sugar problems.
- Fatigue.

You may not experience every one of these symptoms, but if you are low in energy and suffering from general malaise, there is good reason to believe that your liver could be at the root of your problem.

Other detox organs

Also involved in detoxing are your kidneys, colon, lungs, lymphatic system and skin. The kidneys act like a water purifier, filtering out toxins, waste products and excess sodium in your blood, and disposing of it through your urine. They also produce an enzyme that regulates blood pressure and can become overloaded when your diet is high in salt. Similarly, drinking too little fluid concentrates the urine, increasing the risk of stones, which are formed from mineral salts; stones interrupt the filtering mechanism, which means that the kidneys are pressured and less effective at their job.

From the moment you place food in your mouth, your digestive system springs into action, transforming the food into a liquid from which nutrients are absorbed, mostly in the small intestine. Waste material is concentrated in and then passed out from the colon. Just as your liver and kidneys need to be clear and clean to do their job effectively, so must your colon and other parts of your digestive system. Constipation causes the bowel to work slowly and sluggishly. Toxins are effectively trapped, allowing them to putrefy, ferment and possibly be reabsorbed.

This can not only lead to disease, but to the build-up of hard deposits of faeces and also hardened mucus (see page 23). The balance of the colon and gut is affected, with unhealthy bacteria and intestinal parasites fed by putrefying waste. In essence, if your food is not moving efficiently through your system, with toxins being regularly removed through elimination, your health will suffer.

Your lungs are also important for the detoxification process. A polluted environment and poor breathing techniques can reduce the lungs' ability to oxygenate blood and remove carbon dioxide. A lack of oxygen diminishes the working capacity of the liver, kidneys and digestive tract, and too much carbon dioxide poisons the system. The lungs also have a critical role to play, as they are the first detox organ to get in contact with airborne toxins, chemicals, viruses, bacteria and allergens. It is very important, therefore, that we keep our lungs clean and clear and working at optimum level, through exercise, avoiding smoking and pollution, and through healthy breathing (see page 35). Don't underestimate how important they are to your health and detox status.

Your skin is also crucially important to detoxification, and as the largest organ in the body, it plays an important role in excreting salt, water, the nitrogen-containing waste products of metabolism (including ammonia, urea and uric acid) and even heavy metals. The skin also has the ability to transform toxins from lipid-soluble, or oil-based compounds, into water-soluble forms, which can then be removed by the kidneys. It is also able to absorb toxins, which is why it is important to avoid using products that contain chemicals which can cause ill health or lead to toxic overload (see page 11). Your skin can be damaged by overuse of products, and overexposure to the sun, which can cause scarring. It also becomes clogged and less efficient when it is not cleaned properly, and when dead skin cells, oil and dirt, as well as make-up and other personal hygiene products, block the pores.

Your lymphatic system runs parallel to the circulatory system in tiny channels where fluid, known as lymph, collects. This colourless, odourless fluid helps to nourish the body by transporting nutrients, such as salts, proteins and minerals, to every part of your body. Many cells in your body receive their nutrients directly from the lymphatic fluids that surround them. This fluid also gathers together the waste products that the cells produce, and delivers them to the blood, which carries them away for elimination. Protein molecules can block the lymphatic system and lack of exercise can make it sluggish, meaning that it cannot do its job effectively. A diet that is high in fatty or animal protein-rich foods can cause stagnation in the lymphatic system, and recurrent illnesses can cause the lymph nodes – glands scattered throughout the body which help to trap invading disease micro-organisms – to swell, causing further blockages. Undigested food, infectious material, dead cells and other debris have to be carried off by the lymphatic system. Thickened and sluggish lymph results in swelling and discomfort and will affect every organ in your body.

Why detox?

The purpose of detox diets and programmes is multifold. At the outset, the idea is to remove pressure from the liver – ostensibly giving it a rest, and allowing it to rejuvenate and renew itself. By ensuring that your diet and lifestyle are as free from toxins as possible, your liver will become less congested and able to function more easily, which impacts on every other system in the body, and it can then work to heal itself.

Detoxing works because it gives your body a break from the toxic excesses that modern life creates. By removing the body's need to burn energy digesting heavy, sugary, fat-laden meals and snacks that are difficult to metabolise and that play havoc with blood sugar, your energy is released to cleanse and regenerate the body's tissues and vital organs.

It's not just the liver that is involved in detoxification; a good detox programme will also work to cleanse the bowels, kidneys, lymphatic system, lungs and skin, and to encourage healthy elimination and immune function. When these organs and systems are able to do their jobs properly, the liver can perform more efficiently.

It's also important to support the liver, kidneys and digestive system by eating foods and taking herbs that stimulate and heal, encouraging the body's natural ability to deal with toxins and other invaders. When the body is working at optimum level, good health is restored, as are vitality and energy. You can expect to enjoy clearer skin, weight loss (if required) and reduction of water retention, brighter eyes, a stronger immune system, greater mental clarity and even moods, balanced hormones and blood-sugar levels, healthy digestion and elimination and, in a nutshell, relief from all of the symptoms that characterise a sluggish liver.

What does it involve?

Most detoxes are short-term diets, simply because they involve removing some key food groups from your daily diet, which could, over time, result in deficiencies. Having said that, however, there is no reason why the elements of a detox diet can't be incorporated into daily life in the long term. The foods you will be cutting out of your diet will be replaced with others that are bursting with nutritional and health benefits, as well as antioxidants (substances found in our food that help to prevent the damage caused by free radicals and many of the degenerative diseases related to ageing) and other compounds that the body needs for regular, healthy detoxification.

You'll also be eating foods that contain plenty of fibre, such as whole grains and fruit and vegetables, as well as drinking a lot more water, to draw out and eliminate toxins by increasing the frequency of your bowel movements and urination. This encourages the health of the digestive system, which means that the nutrients in your food are much more easily absorbed and assimilated by your body.

Detoxing is not about starving and, in fact, the weight loss that does occur is merely the result of healthier eating habits, more efficient metabolism and digestion and having more energy that will naturally make you more active.

Your diet can also be supplemented with herbs and other dietary aids that will encourage the process of detoxification and improve your health on all levels.

Preparing for a detox

It's important to prepare yourself for a detox – physically, mentally and practically. To begin with, detoxing does cause some symptoms as stored toxins are released and processed. It's rather like cleaning out an old, dirty cupboard! There may, potentially, be years' worth of toxins built up in cells throughout your body and, as they are released, you may feel under the weather (see pages 43–5). Try to see this as a good sign as it shows your body is at work. You may be (or know of) one of those people who seem never to suffer from hangovers no matter how much they drink. That is, in fact, not a good sign; it indicates that the toxins in alcohol aren't being dealt with, merely deposited elsewhere in the body. A healthy liver gets straight to work on toxins such as alcohol, and as they are cleared, your body responds immediately.

So, to make things slightly easier at the outset, it's a good idea to begin with some physical preparation. If you are a big drinker, cut down the week before your detox, and try to go a few days without any alcohol at all. If you drink a lot of coffee, try weaning yourself down to a cup or two a day, and experiment with some of the alternatives, such as green tea, chicory tea or coffee or dandelion root coffee, which enhance rather than detract from health. Do you smoke? Cut down, or take the opportunity to stop. Even the best diet can't negate the impact of the chemicals contained in cigarette smoke, so if you care about your health it's time to address this habit.

Consider beginning a very basic exercise programme to enhance your detox programme (see page 34). If you start moving – even just walking more often and taking the stairs rather than the lift – your circulation will improve, which feeds systems and organs in your body with oxygenated blood, and improves elimination of toxins from the cells. This not only makes your detox more effective and efficient, but also helps to ease symptoms that may crop up.

Emotionally, you may be wary about making changes to your diet and lifestyle, no matter how grim you may have been feeling or how promising the results may appear. There is no doubt that the prospect of dietary changes can be daunting, and giving up your favourite tipple or regular takeaway may be difficult; however, the detox programme is intended to be short term, and you can choose to undertake it for as long as you wish. Even the 24-hour spring-clean (see page 28) can impact on your health and your body's ability to work more efficiently. If you feel that your body has taken a battering over the last few months or years, it may well be time to bite the bullet and go for a longer-term clear-out. Although some sacrifices may need to be made, the positive benefits will begin to show within days, and you may well be inspired to carry on for longer than you had predicted.

The secret to preparing yourself emotionally is to stay positive and to get some support. In the first instance, you can start by writing down what you hope to achieve and what niggling symptoms you wish to banish. Stick this on your fridge, and if you are tempted to reach for a cold glass of wine or a sausage roll, remind yourself what you are doing and why. It can also help to keep a diary, noting down any positive changes you experience – such as brighter eyes, more regular bowel movements, increased energy, deeper and more restful sleep, and having an even temper. Read through this regularly to reinforce your desire to continue.

Detoxing with a friend or partner can also help to make the process easier – and more fun. If there is more than one of you abstaining from unhealthy treats, another pair of hands to prepare some of the dishes and some emotional support when the going gets tough, you will be much more likely to succeed. Take time, too, to pamper yourself a little – indulge in steamy baths with delicious detoxifying essential oils (see page 68) or treat yourself to a massage, which can get things moving. Invest in a juicer and replace your usual fizzy drinks or cocktails with wonderful blends of nourishing, cleansing fruit and vegetable juices. Consider purchasing a few new organic body and face creams to nourish from the outside in, as your detox works its magic inside.

Being prepared in a practical way also makes the job that much more straightforward. Clear your fridge and cupboards of foods that are off the menu, and replace them with healthy, fresh ingredients. Take time to visit a farmer's market or an organic greengrocer to get the best fresh produce you can find, and experiment with some of the exciting recipes that appear later in this book. Prepare some of the snacks and meals in advance, so you won't be tempted to get a takeaway or rush to the nearest sandwich bar to fill an empty tummy, and keep a good supply of healthy, detox snacks to hand, wherever you are. Look through the list of menu ideas, and make a note of the ingredients that you'll need to prepare some of the recipes. And fill your fridge to bursting with any of the detox superfoods listed later in the book (see page 82). Each of these will play a role in encouraging the health of your liver, kidneys and other detox organs and, in most cases (with a few exceptions; see the lists on pages 33–4 and 41–2), they can be eaten in unlimited quantities. Purchase some airtight containers so that you can take food with you when you are on the move and invest in a steamer, which allows you to preserve the most nutrients when you cook your meals.

More personally, it's well worth investing in a skin brush with natural bristles, as well as some exfoliating salts or creams, to practise some dry skin brushing (see page 73) and encourage the process of elimination. On page 68, you'll also find some great essential oils as well as herbs, homoeopathic remedies and supplements, which can be purchased in advance to support the detoxification process along with your liver and other organs.

Foods to avoid

A good detox programme focuses on removing foods that put pressure on your liver, kidneys and other detoxification organs. Some are toxic, such as coffee, alcohol and preservatives; others, such as fatty foods, simply make a great deal more work for the liver and digestive system, and slow down the process of elimination.

The foods listed on pages 20–6 should not appear in your diet for the duration of your detox. Instead, you'll be including healthy, nourishing and nutritious foods that actively encourage the process of detoxification and elimination, and the health of your liver and other detox organs. In fact, you will be delighted and surprised to see the number of foods that are on the menu – delicious goodies that will tempt even the fussiest eater! But before we go any further, let's take a look at what is definitely off the list.

Alcohol

Alcohol is the most common chemical responsible for toxic damage to the liver, causing fatty liver, alcoholic hepatitis and eventually cirrhosis, which is life-threatening. Much of the cell damage that occurs during liver degeneration is believed to be caused by free radicals, highly reactive molecular fragments liberated during alcohol metabolism. The damage caused by free radicals can include the destruction of essential components of cell membranes. Alcohol also kills off cells and alters critical parts of the brain, leading to impairment of thinking and structural brain changes. It harms the kidneys by raising blood pressure, which is a leading cause of kidney disease, as well as by damaging the nephrons, the functioning units of the kidneys which filter the blood.

Artificial additives

Artificial additives are chemicals which are added to foods, and include colourings, flavourings, emulsifiers, stabilisers, preservatives, fillers, sweeteners, flavour enhancers and antioxidants (the latter added to preserve the food – not to be confused with naturally occurring antioxidants, which are found in fruits and vegetables, such as vitamins A, C and E). Every chemical that enters our body has to be detoxified by the liver, and the additives contained in the food we eat put considerable strain on this organ, as well as other body systems. Some are toxic in large quantities, and when the body can't remove them, they are stored – where they are free to cause damage.

Coffee, tea and other caffeine-containing drinks

Firstly, coffee is one of the most heavily pesticide-sprayed crops in the world, and every cup you drink means exposure to those chemicals.

Secondly, there is plenty of evidence showing that heavy coffee drinkers are much more likely to get type 2 diabetes, which suggests that a chemical contained within coffee has a negative effect on blood sugar and insulin production; indeed, coffee artificially raises blood sugar, giving you a burst of energy followed by a slump. There are literally hundreds of chemicals in coffee, many of which have not been scientifically analysed, and their impact on health is unknown. What we do know is that the caffeine in coffee is linked to infertility, breast cancer, hormonal imbalance, high blood pressure and osteoporosis.

Tea isn't much better, really. It's high in caffeine, which acts in the same way as that in coffee, and unless you always drink organic tea, you'll be getting a host of unpleasant chemicals, including fungicides, pesticides and herbicides. What's more, tea plants that are treated with nitrogen fertilisers have a 40 per cent higher caffeine content.

Coffee and tea do both have some health benefits, however, and may be drunk in small quantities in daily life – but they have no place in a detox diet. For one thing, they are both powerful diuretics, which can rob the body of key vitamins and minerals. There are some foods and drinks that are natural diuretics, which help to cleanse the kidneys; however, these are gentle, and naturally support the action of the kidneys rather than overworking them. Drinking plenty of water is the best way to prevent dehydration.

Caffeine occurs in both tea and coffee, as well as cola drinks and even chocolate, so these should not appear on your detox programme. The one exception is green tea (see page 118), which does contain a little caffeine, but also has health benefits that far outweigh the dangers.

Dairy products

Dairy products are off the list, mainly because they promote the build-up of mucus, which can hamper digestive function and assimilation. Furthermore, because of modern factory farming methods and the levels of pesticides used in farming, dairy products contain residues of the pesticides used in growing the grain that is fed to cows, as well as the hormones and antibiotics given directly to the animals. These residues accumulate in reproductive organs and in the cow's udder. For these reasons, dairy products increase your levels of toxicity, which is counterproductive during a detox and puts additional strain on your liver. Finally, about 75 per cent of the population have difficulty digesting cow's milk because of the sugar it contains, known as lactose. As we get older, the ability to digest lactose diminishes, and we can suffer a number of symptoms. Lactose intolerance can cause gastric upset, which in turn causes stomach irritation and a leaky intestinal barrier that places a heavy load on the liver detox system.

'Diet' or 'low-cal' foods

Low-fat, low-calorie and 'diet' foods are designed by manufacturers to satisfy the taste buds without offering the usual levels of fat. However, in order to do so, they often rely on additives and chemicals to ensure that the consistency remains similar to the original product and that it is high in flavour. So, rather than fat, you'll find things like MSG (monosodium glutamate), emulsifiers, flavour enhancers, artificial sweeteners or sugar and other chemical additives that will do nothing to encourage overall health, will probably play havoc with your blood-sugar levels and also place pressure on your liver. What's more, many contain trans fats, which are very detrimental to health, causing heart disease, obesity and other health problems. So leave all 'diet' foods and drinks off the menu for the duration of the detox.

Fatty foods

Some fats are not only healthy but absolutely essential. However, foods that contain high levels of saturated fats (which means they are solid at room temperature) are most definitely off limits. For one thing, animal fats, such as dairy produce and meat, can be toxic to the liver, creating a high workload for both the liver and the gall bladder. Second to this is the fact that the liver is the main fat-burning organ in the body, and is responsible for removing fatty acids from the bloodstream and regulating both fat and carbohydrate metabolism. A diet that is high in saturated fats puts a strain on the liver, which is what you'll be aiming to avoid during your detox. In fact, one sign of a fatty liver (see page 11) is an inability to tolerate fatty foods, which indicates that your liver is overloaded and unable to cope. By taking the pressure off during your detox, you'll encourage your liver to heal and clear out stored toxins.

What do we mean by fatty foods? Dairy produce (see above), deep-fried and fried foods, margarines, processed vegetable oils (hydrogenated fats, known as trans fats), preserved meats, skin on meat or poultry and all fatty meats.

Meat and poultry

For the same reason that fatty foods are off the menu, it's important to avoid meat and poultry, because animal fats (even lean ones), work to clog the liver and put it under pressure. Moreover, when meat is cooked, carcinogens are produced. In most cases, the body and, in particular the liver, can deal with these; however, a high intake of meat and poultry, combined with a liver that is struggling, can increase your risk of cancer, in particular of colon cancer.

Meat and poultry are also known as 'acid-forming' foods, which increase mucus in the body and are responsible for the development of 'mucoid plaque', which is hardened mucus that traps debris in the colon and prevents healthy digestion, elimination and gut health. The protein structure of most meats is much more complex and harder to digest than that of plants, which puts an enormous strain on the liver as partially digested protein molecules enter the bloodstream and must effectively be eliminated from the blood.

Finally, unless you eat entirely organic meat and poultry, you will be getting a dose of whatever the animal in question was dosed with – growth enhancers, antibiotics, the pesticides and herbicides used on their food and even hormones. After your detox, meat and poultry are fine in moderation (about two servings a week is enough, if you balance them with healthy vegetable proteins), but always choose organic if possible.

Potatoes

Although there is nothing wrong with the humble potato, which does provide a wealth of nutrients and even a little protein, it will not feature in the *Perfect Detox*, and here's why. First of all, potatoes are a high GI food, which is linked to fatty liver disease (see page 11). In a nutshell, this means that the starch in potatoes is converted to sugar and enters the bloodstream very quickly after eating, which puts pressure on the liver. What's more, high potato consumption is linked to diabetes. Although potatoes do contain decent amounts of other nutrients, their high natural starch content means that they should not be a daily feature of your post-detox diet, either. Unless you are lean and very active, potatoes will provide you with a whack of glucose that can upset your blood-sugar levels and lead to health problems.

Ready meals and sauces

Ready meals, whether they are fresh or frozen, contain preservatives and other additives that allow them to stay fresh for longer and to taste appealing. They tend to contain high levels of salt and/or sugar, as well as saturated fat. They also fall under the umbrella of 'processed food', which means that they have, in many cases, had most of their nutrients stripped from them. Moreover, they have often been pre-cooked and then require more cooking in the reheating process, which effectively destroys most of the nutrients they contain. Don't be fooled by the 'good for you' hype of so-called 'healthier' ready meals. While an effort may have been made to reduce salt, sugar and fat, the chemical load is likely to be much the same if not greater, and can undermine any progress you make on your detox diet.

For much the same reason that ready meals are not appropriate for your detox diet, ready-bought sauces and condiments should also be avoided. They tend to be high in sugar, salt, saturated fat or trans fats, as well as artificial ingredients to ensure they do not lose their 'fresh-ness'. They are often heat-treated for the same reason, which destroys any nutrients they may contain. You are aiming to reduce all unnatural chemicals on your detox diet, and that means excluding foods that contain them. Fortunately, it's easy to make healthy, fresh and nutritious meals and sauces from the foods you can eat on the detox diet. See pages 123–57 for recipes.

Salt

A small amount of salt is important for good health, as it helps to maintain the correct volume of circulating blood and tissue fluids in the body. Our kidneys are the main salt regulators in our bodies and too much salt can put enormous pressure on them, leading to kidney stones and poor function. This affects the way the body eliminates waste in the form of urine, which can pose even more problems. Many of us have overeaten salt for years; in fact, on average, we eat about ten times the amount we actually need. Your *Perfect Detox* diet aims to cut out salt almost completely (with only a little natural sea salt, which is high in hormone-balancing iodine, being used in some recipes; see under 'Seaweed', page 115), to take the pressure off your kidneys and reduce the fluid retention that may be discouraging your body from working efficiently. When we say 'cut out salt' we mean all foods containing it, too, such as sauces, snacks, baked goods and even tinned vegetables.

Sugar and refined carbs

Sugar and refined carbohydrates not only play havoc with blood-sugar levels, which puts pressure on your liver, but research indicates that they are the one of the greatest causes of fatty liver disease (see page 11), which can severely compromise liver function. Sugar that is released by high GI foods, such as potatoes, white bread, white rice and pasta, as well as anything made from white flour or sugar, encourages the production of the hormone insulin, which tells the body to make and store fat. This message is strongest in the liver, where insulin concentrations can be many times higher than in the rest of the body. Research has found that these raised insulin levels can lead to a build-up of fat in the liver which may be severe enough to cause harm, and which may have no symptoms until it is too late. Many studies have also linked sugar with reduced immunity (just a few teaspoons can reduce immunity by 25 per cent, for example). What's more, sugar and high-sugar foods encourage the proliferation of unhealthy bacteria in the gut, which means poor elimination of toxins and other waste, as well as reduced assimilation of nutrients. Watch out for sugar in everything you eat; you'll find it in many savoury foods as well as sweet. Avoid adding it to anything you cook or eat on the *Perfect Detox* diet.

Wheat

On its own, wheat is a nutritious grain in its whole form; however, not only do we tend to overeat wheat in the West, but we also tend to use refined forms which have virtually no nutritional value whatsoever. Research indicates that as many as one-third of us have a sensitivity to wheat – mainly because our bodies have not adapted to the introduction of wheat (particularly at such high levels) in our diets. Wheat also has a complex structure that is hard to digest, and most of us fail to absorb a large percentage of the starch it contains. These starches are then fermented by the bacteria in the gut, which produces gases and acids that damage the lining. By giving up wheat for the duration of your detox, and even beyond if you can, you'll encourage the gut to heal, which will ensure it can efficiently assimilate nutrients as well as eliminate toxins successfully.

The one exception to the no-wheat rule is wheatgrass, which was once a staple food of our ancestors, and which contains a huge range of vitamins and minerals as well as enzymes that promote healthy digestion, antioxidants and amino acids (the building blocks of protein). The high chlorophyll content of wheatgrass juice causes increased haemoglobin production in the body, which in turn encourages the blood to carry more oxygen. The benefits of highly oxygenated blood include purification of the blood, improvement in blood-sugar disorders, and the more efficient detoxification of carbon monoxide, cigarette smoke and heavy metals. Wheatgrass is also a great source of fibre, which can help maintain bowel health.

A word about eggs ...

Some detox programmes ban eggs. However, eggs are a perfectly healthy, balanced and pure form of protein and other nutrients, and they are rich in sulphur, which is particularly good for the liver by assisting the process of producing bile. What's more, they contain high levels of lethicin, which is a fat emulsifier. Choose free-range or organic eggs that have added omega 3, for extra benefits. For those of you who have been brought up on the notion that eggs cause high cholesterol, rest assured that this theory has been discredited. Unless you've been diagnosed as a hyper-responder to cholesterol, eggs are a nutritious and cleansing addition to any detox diet.

Getting started

The benefits of detoxing are limitless, and you can expect to feel better on all levels – fresher, brighter and full of energy, as your body works more efficiently and effectively. That's not to say that the process is easy. You may experience side-effects somewhere along the line (see pages 43–5), and you may also find that it can be difficult to make a massive adjustment to your lifestyle, even in the short term. For this reason, we've come up with a few different ways to approach your *Perfect Detox*. Let's examine them now.

2 Your detox plan

Perfect Detox is designed to be flexible, and you can adapt it to work according to what you feel you need from the programme. You can choose a 24-hour detox and repeat it as required, or you can dig your heels in and detox for a week or even a fortnight. We don't recommend that you detox for longer than two weeks at a time, as you may miss out on some important food groups that are essential to health, but our 30-day plan will keep you well nourished while clearing out your system over a longer period of time, and we have plenty of tips for maintaining the effects of your detox long after you have finished the programme.

In the previous chapter we looked at the foods you need to avoid, and the reasons why this is necessary. While it can seem daunting to give up favourite foods or tipples, the good news is that you will soon adjust to your new lifestyle, and probably won't even miss them. And if you slip, there are some tried-and-tested tricks to get you back on track. What's more, there is a multitude of healthy, delicious foods on the menu, and we've come up with some inventive, mouth-watering recipes to help you incorporate them into your new rich and varied diet.

For now, however, let's look at the programmes on offer, and work out what you need to do to get your detox under way.

24-hour detox

As a short-term fix, our 24-hour detox can be a good way to brush out some of the cobwebs and toxins, and take the pressure off your system. Anyone will benefit from this programme, but it's particularly useful if you've had a period of heavy partying, stress, an inadequate diet and exposure to chemicals. The 24-hour detox is enough to give your body a boost of key nutrients and clear out debris. It isn't a long-term solution to an overtaxed liver or other detox organs, but it will cleanse your body and revitalise you. If a longer detox isn't possible, undertaking a 24-hour detox just once a week or fortnight can have a long-lasting impact on your health and energy levels.

Some experts recommend fresh juices only for a 24-hour detox, and while these definitely give you a good dose of easily digested nutrients, and take the pressure off your digestive system, they don't work to cleanse in the same way that the *Perfect Detox* 24-hour plan does. We suggest plenty of cleansing fibre, to clear out your colon and stimulate your liver function. We also suggest foods that will offer specific cleansing benefits, and provide protection from toxins in your diet and lifestyle.

What does it involve?

You'll start your day with a mug of warm, not hot, water, with the juice of a lemon. If the water is too hot or too cold then it will cause the body to expend energy in order to process it. Lemon water cleanses and stimulates the liver and kidneys, and acts as an antiseptic to the entire digestive system.

Wait an hour, and then have a big bowl of fresh porridge, made with rolled oats that you've left to soak overnight. Top with as many fresh berries as you can, a swirl of Manuka honey (see page 101), which has impressive antibacterial action, and a handful of raw almonds.

Mid-morning, have another glass of warm lemon water and the seeds from a fresh pomegranate.

Lunch will consist of a bowl of steamed brown rice, which will act as a broom to clean out your digestive system; top with steamed green vegetables (choose any you like from the detox superfoods at the end of the book; see pages 82–122). If you prefer your veggies raw, all the better! Top with a scattering of chickpeas, and then season with a little lemon juice, olive oil and any fresh herbs that tickle your fancy. We like chervil,

Can I fast instead?

Many experts recommend regular fasting for 24-hour periods, to cleanse the body and kick-start your metabolism and body functions. There is no reason why a short-term fast, with plenty of liquids to nourish and hydrate, can't work, but fasting for longer than this can be dangerous, upsetting blood-sugar levels, causing vitamin and mineral deficiency and leading to muscle breakdown. If you are tempted to fast, choose nutritious juices, such as carrot, apple, melon, beet, watercress and cucumber, which will keep things ticking over, and do not fast for longer than 24 hours. In reality, our 24-hour detox will be much more effective, because it actively works to remove toxins from your body.

chives and mint, but dill, basil, thyme and parsley are also great, and parsley in particular is a great detox aid.

Mid-afternoon, have another glass of warm lemon water, and a sliced apple with the skin left on. If you are feeling peckish, a handful of raw walnuts will do the trick.

Dinner will be a big bowl of steamed brown rice, with a little organic natural soy sauce. Top with as many brightly coloured vegetables as you can, such as carrots, butternut squash, kale, yellow peppers or broccoli.

Before bed, drink a cup of warm chamomile tea with a slice of lemon.

Top tips

- Choose a period when you have no other commitments, and can focus on the programme.
- Aim to drink seven or eight large glasses of water throughout the day, preferably mineral water in a glass bottle (not plastic, which leaches chemicals into the water). Lukewarm is easiest on the digestion.
- Chew your food carefully, concentrating on every mouthful. Studies show that every spoonful should be chewed at least 20 times, and if it doesn't seem liquid at that point, chew some more! The action of

chewing mechanically breaks down very large aggregates of food molecules into smaller particles. This results in the food having an increased surface area, an important contributing factor to good digestion. Digestion also begins in the mouth with enzymes in saliva breaking down the food. If you bolt it, none of this happens.

- Take one 45-minute walk (or, if you are a regular runner, jog) mid-morning.
- Before bed, practise a relaxation exercise (see page 79), followed by a warm bath with one or two of the best detoxifying essential oils (see page 68). Before you get into the steaming tub, dry brush your skin to get the circulation and lymphatic system working efficiently (see page 73).
- Don't eat anything other than what has been suggested. If you feel hungry, have a cup of dandelion-root coffee or some nettle tea instead.
- If you've got some time on your hands, pay a visit to a massage therapist for some deep-tissue cleansing, or visit a steam room or sauna, which will encourage detoxification through your skin.
- If you are a smoker, try to give up for 24 hours. If that's impossible, cut down as much as possible, and pop 100mg of vitamin C for every cigarette you take.

Maintenance

Once you've started the process of detoxing, you may well be inclined to continue. In this case, head straight for our 14-day programme, and get things really moving. If it's going to prove difficult at the moment, why not cut out a few key foods that tend to place pressure on the body? You could:

- Give up dairy and all other animal produce (apart from live yoghurt; see page 121) for a week or two.
- Try to aim for at least eight detox superfoods each day, spread between three meals and two snacks.
- Limit yourself to one alcoholic drink a week (if you find this hard, just make sure you never drink more than one drink a day).

- Incorporate as many raw foods into your diet as you can.
- Cut out every food in your diet that isn't whole or natural – so give junk food, prepared foods and condiments a miss for as long as you can.
- Try to eat at least three fruits or vegetables raw every day.
- Add brown rice to your diet at least once a day. Not only does it sweep out debris from your digestive system, but it's also a rich source of vitamins and minerals (see page 114), and you'll soon experience the benefits.
- Start taking some supplements – herbal, nutritional or otherwise – to support and nourish your detox organs. Even if you have a diet that is less than perfect, and imbibe more than you would like to, these supplements can help to balance and prevent toxins from becoming stored, rather than excreted.
- Use aromatherapy oils and other detox aids as often as you can, to keep things moving in the right direction, and take the pressure off your system. See Detox Aids, pages 57–81.

14-day detox

A 14-day detox will give your body a deeper clean and actively work to remove toxins, as well as providing support for the organs involved in detoxifying. You'll need to avoid all of the foods and drinks listed on pages 20–6, and aim to include as many of our detox superfoods as possible, creating a varied, balanced diet with the full spectrum of nutrients. You'll be getting plenty of healthy calories on this programme, so you shouldn't feel hungry; you may, however, experience some symptoms associated with detoxing, particularly in the early days (see pages 43–5).

What does it involve?

Every morning you'll begin your day with a cup of warm water and lemon juice (see page 103), to set things in motion. If you are a coffee addict, you may wish to follow this with a cup of dandelion-root coffee (no milk or sugar, please) or, if a cup of tea is your usual eye-opener, choose green tea which is rich in flavonoids (see page 118). Wait for at least 30 minutes after finishing your lemon water before eating.

You'll be eating three meals every day, with a snack between meals. If you tend to graze rather than eat full meals, you can eat little and often throughout the day, breaking down the suggested meals into smaller parcels. Always stop eating when you are satisfied, and try not to add anything else to your menu.

Every day you will need to include:

- Three to five servings of complex carbohydrates, remembering that wheat is not on the menu for the duration of your detox; one of these must be a bowl of steamed brown rice. We suggest organic brown basmati or short-grain brown rice. Other good choices include oats, wild rice, quinoa, barley or millet. For recipe ideas, see pages 123–57.
- Three servings of good-quality protein from vegetable sources, such as lentils, beans, tofu, peas and chickpeas.
- At least two servings of cooked vegetables from the detox superfood list.
- At least three servings of raw vegetables from the detox superfood list (salad vegetables are fine).
- At least three servings of fresh or dried fruit from the detox superfood list.
- Two handfuls of raw nuts from the detox superfood list.
- Two handfuls of raw seeds from the detox superfood list.
- 125ml fresh organic plain live yoghurt.
- Unlimited caffeine-free herbal teas, lemon water, freshly squeezed fruit and vegetable juices, dandelion-root coffee and at least eight glasses of natural mineral water.
- One multi-vitamin and mineral supplement.
- Psyllium husks and seeds, which must usually be soaked before eating.
- One or two detox supplements of your choice – if this is your first time detoxing, take uva ursi for your kidneys and milk thistle to

promote the health of your liver; you may choose to take a detox blend, so look out for one that contains any of the remedies suggested in Detox Aids (pages 57–81).

- One probiotic supplement, particularly if you aren't able to eat live yoghurt.
- In addition, aim for three servings of fish each week, preferably oily fish such as fresh tuna, mackerel or salmon, as well as two eggs.

Lifestyle

Food isn't the only important element of a detox diet. In addition to altering your diet to include three meals and two snacks based on the above, you'll also need to undertake at least 45 minutes of exercise a day. Equally important is relaxing properly, getting plenty of good, restful sleep, and looking after your skin, which you may be surprised to learn plays a very important role in the detoxificatin process.

Exercise

Exercise has a host of health benefits, and will encourage the process of detoxification. For one thing, exercise requires energy, and will call upon stores of body fat to keep you going. This is very important in the process of detoxing, as toxins are stored in fats and exercise will encourage their release into the bloodstream, from where they can eventually be excreted from your body.

Another of the key benefits of exercise is increased blood and lymph circulation. Your blood and lymphatic fluids distribute essential nutrients to your cells and remove metabolic waste and other toxic substances from them. So not only will you be stimulating these two important systems, encouraging the flow of nutrients and oxygen to the cells and that of waste products and toxins away from them, but you will be exercising your lungs, which are another important way that the body eliminates toxins.

And there is more! Regular exercise has been linked to a lower risk of breast cancer and an improved immune system. It helps to keep your bowels working efficiently, which means you are eliminating waste products your body doesn't need. It stimulates your thyroid gland and

A note about breathing

The lungs are important detox organs, and they should be exercised to make them more efficient. It is always a good idea to breathe in through your nose, which provides a filter for toxins from the outside world. Breathing directly through your mouth into your lungs puts more pressure on these key organs, as they are then in direct contact with any toxins or contaminants such as pollution, bacteria, viruses and even pollen.

helps to improve thyroid function, which has a direct effect on your metabolism. Physical exercise improves your ability to sleep soundly, because the brain compensates for physical stress by increasing deep sleep. Exercise also revitalises the nervous system, activates the endocrine system (hormones) and eases muscular tension, all of which encourage healthy sleep patterns. Exercise reduces stress by using up the adrenaline that is created by stress and stressful situations. It also creates endorphins, the 'feel-good' hormones that improve mood, motivation and even tolerance to pain and other stimuli.

If you aren't regularly active, it's absolutely fine to start by walking. Your aim will be to hit 10,000 steps a day over the coming weeks, starting with about 3,000 to 4,000 if you aren't particularly fit, and adding 500 steps every three days until you reach the target. You'll need to purchase a pedometer, which will give you an idea of how many steps you are achieving now, and allow you to keep track easily. Increase your daily steps by taking the stairs instead of the lift, walking part of the way to work, parking as far away as possible from your destination, taking the dog for a walk or meeting up with friends for a power walk.

What about pace? Aim to become breathless, and get your heart and lungs working to the point that you are still able to talk without gasping for breath. If you don't have time for the step challenge, then at least aim for a 30-minute walk every day.

Other good forms of exercise include jogging, swimming, cycling, trampolining, or playing football, tennis, badminton or basketball.

Many people find it easier to get involved in team sports, as they normally have to make a commitment to be there.

Try abdominal exercises. You may wish to hit the gym to get your abs working. The idea here is not to produce a perfectly flat tummy, but to work the core muscles. This helps to maintain the health of your key elimination organs (colon, kidneys and liver), and helps to stimulate and strengthen the muscles around them, which makes them more efficient.

Try some ordinary stomach crunches: lie on your back, with your knees bent and your feet flat on the floor. Lift yourself up and off the ground, reaching your elbows to your knees. After 10 repetitions, reach your elbows to the opposite knee – so your right elbow to your left knee, and vice versa. This produces a 'twisting' effect that stimulates the muscles of the colon, which in turn encourages elimination and blood supply to the area. If you are very unfit, you may only manage a few, but adding five more repetitions a day will soon help you to reach a target of 50 repetitions per day. If you are superfit, do as many as you can.

Any other exercise you choose to do above and beyond this will be a bonus, but be aware that you may feel a bit unwell during the first few days of exercising. This is no excuse to avoid it, as the act of exercising will lift your spirits as well as improving symptoms by getting things moving in your body, and giving your cells fresh, oxygenated blood. But if you find it difficult and you are suffering from withdrawal symptoms from some of your favourite foods (such as refined carbs, which can leave you feeling a bit weak for a day or two), take it easy, and make sure you stop at any point if you experience dizziness or discomfort.

Caring for your skin

Every other day you should dry-brush your skin (see page 73) to keep it clean, clear and stimulated. If the idea of a salt bath doesn't appeal, go for a hot bath with a few drops of detoxifying essential oils, which will help to draw out the toxins, as well as directly affect key detox organs. Choose a moisturiser to hydrate your skin following your bath; light oils such as rose or orange blossom help to seal in moisture and hydrate, while allowing your skin to 'breathe' and expel toxins.

It's also a good idea to take a hot shower in the morning, using a loofah or organic flannel to gently exfoliate your skin. Finish off with a blast of cold water, which will increase circulation, tone skin and muscles and leave you feeling invigorated.

Choose natural and organic skin products, if possible, which will nurture your skin and support its natural actions; detoxing your body from the inside out is bound to be less effective if you are slathering chemicals on to the outside! There is a huge number of organic products now available, containing herbs, essential oils, essential fatty acids, antioxidants, vitamins and minerals, which are absorbed into the bloodstream, providing a boost to every system in the body.

Some of the things you *don't* want to find in your skincare products include:

- **Mineral oils and petrolatum**: derived from petroleum, they block pores and diminish the skin's ability to function.
- **Sodium lauryl sulphate** (SLS): a detergent that can irritate the skin, and destroy skin and eye proteins.
- **Sodium laureth sulphate** (SLES): a foaming agent that can leave traces of cancer-causing residues.
- **TEA** (Triethanolamine): used to control pH, this can break down to form cancer-causing nitrosamine chemicals.
- **Quaternium-15**: used as a preservative, it can be contaminated with cancer-causing impurities, and can trigger an immune response including itching, burning, scaling, hives and blistering.
- **Parfum**: a fancy name for fragrance; can include over 700 chemicals used to make a single fragrance ingredient. A typical shampoo fragrance is, for example, created by mixing up to 100 of these chemicals together. Linked to immune and nervous system toxicity, cancer and reduced fertility.
- **Parabens**: a family of chemicals including methyl paraben, ethyl paraben, etc, may be linked to breast cancer, and are considered 'gender-benders', which affect male fertility and can cause testicular cancer, as well as upsetting hormonal balance in everyone.
- **Lauramide DEA**: a foaming ingredient, linked with cancer in animals.

- **PEG**: an emulsifier linked with cancer.
- **Cocamidopropyl betaine**: a foaming ingredient linked with cancer and dermatitis.
- **AHAs** (glycolic acid): used to exfoliate the skin, and linked with severe immune system responses (including itching, burning and blistering) as well as altering the structure of the skin, making it more susceptible to chemicals and cancer-causing UV rays.
- **Diazolidinyl urea**: a preservative that works by slowly releasing formaldehyde, a known carcinogen. Also toxic to liver and kidneys.

At least one relaxation exercise per day

This will not only produce a feeling of calm, but will help you to focus positively on your body, which can make the whole programme more effective. Our bodies work more efficiently when they are in a relaxed state, and can begin the process of regeneration rather than simply fire-fighting. There are plenty of relaxing exercise programmes you can choose from, including yoga, Pilates and t'ai chi, and you can use meditation or the relaxation exercise suggested on page 79, to restore peace to mind and body.

Sleep

Sleep is absolutely essential for your detox programme, as it plays a number of roles in health – the most important of which is to offer the opportunity to regenerate and revitalise. Burning the candle at both ends puts pressure on every body system, making them all less efficient and effective.

Tips for restful sleep:

- Eat an early dinner so your body can finish the process of digestion before bed.
- Drink herbal tea before bed. Relaxing teas such as chamomile, passionflower, valerian, catnip and skullcap are best.
- Avoid exercise or work-related activities immediately before bed.
- Sprinkle lavender oil on your pillow, which has been proven in several different studies to promote healthy, restful sleep.

- Go to bed at the same time every night.
- Make sure your bedroom is completely dark, as light stimulates the pineal gland which can encourage you to feel more alert.
- Concentrate on breathing deeply and steadily.
- Tense and relax each of your muscles in turn, starting from your toes and working your way up to the top of your head (see page 79).
- Naps during the day are fine if you can sleep well at night. If not, avoid them; they will only exacerbate your sleeping problems.
- Spend 10–15 minutes outside when you get out of bed. This helps reset your day/night clock so your body knows when to sleep.

Supporting the process

Any of the detox aids in chapter 4 will help you on your way, and you should feel free to experiment with different therapies and remedies, including homeopathic remedies and flower essences. Unless you choose a pre-blended multi-herb product, it's probably not a good idea to use more than two or three at a time. Everyone will benefit from a good EFA supplement, and we recommend that you take a good-quality multi-vitamin and mineral tablet throughout the programme, both to ensure that you get all the nutrients you need, and also to make up for any trace deficiencies that may be causing your body to operate below par.

Top tips

All of the tips suggested in our 24-hour detox are relevant here; you may, however, also wish to consider the following:

- Detoxing too quickly can lead to unpleasant symptoms (see pages 43–5), so if you've been pushing yourself, eating the wrong foods and drinking or smoking too much for a long period of time, it makes sense to take it slowly. Eat regularly to keep your blood-sugar levels stable, and drink lots of fresh water to flush out the nasties.
- Stock up well in advance of your programme, and make sure you have the foods and drinks you need to hand. Your cupboards should contain brown rice and quinoa, not chocolate biscuits!

- Get prepared. Cut up fresh crudités and chill them in a little water in the fridge for instant snacks. You could also purchase mini-packets of unsalted raw nuts, seeds and dried fruit (unsulphured, if possible). Similarly, little pots of hummus or tzaziki (see page 152) are definitely on your detox diet, as long as they don't contain any ingredients on the no-no list (see pages 20–6).

- For more substantial instant meals, make up some soups and other dishes in advance, and pop them in the fridge or freezer.

- Choose a wide variety of different fresh fruits and vegetables, grains, pulses and herbs so that you can produce tempting, delicious meals. No one is going to feel inspired by a pile of unappetising, uncooked vegetables. Plan your meals in advance, and make sure you have lots of foods to create sumptuous, satisfying meals.

- Remember that cravings will always pass if you wait long enough. Some foods, such as refined carbohydrates, caffeine, sugar and alcohol can be addictive, and you may experience some discomfort or longing for them at the outset. Try to distract yourself by doing some physical activity, or make a delicious detox snack and settle down with a good book.

- Get some help from the experts – book yourself in for a relaxing, rejuvenating massage or an acupuncture treatment. See a homoeopath, herbalist or aromatherapist who can provide you with remedies that are just right for you, and offer you emotional and physical support throughout the programme.

- Believe in yourself. Any lifestyle change can be difficult to contemplate, let alone undertake, but every little change you make towards good health will reward you in the long run. Even short-term detoxes can be a step in the right direction.

- Reward yourself! Don't consider a detox programme to be some sort of punishment or purgatory. Reward yourself with delicious meals, nurturing therapies and plenty of healthy relaxation. Buy yourself a good book, rent a series of DVDs, sign up for an exercise class or begin a new hobby. Making changes to your lifestyle during the programme can make it easier to make dietary and exercise changes as well, so take advantage of the opportunity.

Maintenance

When you do begin to eat normally again, introduce the foods that you have cut out one by one, so that you can be aware of how your body reacts to each one.

You may find that your digestion is much more efficient, and that sticking to the principles of the *Perfect Detox* programme works well for you. You may find that animal meats, milk and other products make you feel sluggish, and that refined carbohydrates cause blood-sugar fluctuations and cravings that you no longer enjoy. Keeping these foods to a minimum, and exploring the other varied options on offer, can help to sustain the vitality you experience as a result of your *Perfect Detox*.

It is perfectly possible and acceptable to continue to take the supplements for longer than your detox programme. In some cases, herbs and other nutrients can take several months to work, and they can be useful to support you in times of stress, or when your diet or lifestyle are less than ideal.

30-day detox

A slower, gentler programme may be more appropriate for you, particularly if you are feeling very 'toxic' and need to make adjustments over time. A 30-day detox will be more thorough, and have a longer-lasting impact on your health; however, it is a bigger commitment, and you must be prepared for that.

What does it involve?

Follow the principles of the 14-day programme, with the following adjustments:

- You can increase your weekly intake of eggs to four, and also add one serving per week of lean red meat or poultry if you are a meat eater. If you are a vegetarian, or wish to continue on a vegetarian menu, add a B-complex vitamin supplement daily.

- Make sure you have at least two servings of leafy green vegetables per day, and at least one serving of dried fruit – preferably apricots – as well as lots of whole grains and pulses. This will help to make sure you get adequate iron in your diet. Eating these alongside foods rich in vitamin C, such as fresh fruit and vegetables and their juices, will ensure that the iron from your food is assimilated.
- Increase your serving of plain live yoghurt to 250g, and make sure you get at least one 50g serving of tofu or 200ml unsweetened soya milk every day. You can also add some non-cow's milk dairy produce once or twice a week – a little goat's or sheep's cheese or yoghurt, for example. This ensures that your calcium needs are met.
- Give yourself a once-a-week treat, to help sustain you! A small bar of good-quality dark chocolate, some dark-chocolate-covered raisins or brazil nuts, and even a glass of red wine may be just what you need to keep you going, and all of these have some health-giving properties. Don't be tempted to have more, however, as they will undermine your efforts if you overindulge. If you've managed fine without alcohol, don't be tempted to revert; find another indulgence instead!
- Dry-skin brush once a week, rather than every other day.
- Carry on with your supplements; you are very likely to notice a big change, as they can take several weeks to get to work.

Adapting the programmes

You can, of course, undertake your *Perfect Detox* over any time frame, although it's not recommended for longer than 30 days and you shouldn't detox long-term without following a menu plan that ensures you get all the nutrients you need.

You can go on to the 14-day programme for a few days here and there, and then take a break; or try 30 days then take 30 days off before starting again. It's possible to undertake the 14-day programme for a week, but the effects may not be as dramatic. There are most certainly other ways to practise a detox, and you may find that some programmes claim to clear you out in a week. Many of these are too extreme for the average person and less likely to lead to sustainable changes in your diet and lifestyle. They can also leave you at risk of nutritional deficiencies.

The *Perfect Detox* programme is balanced and carefully designed to ensure that you get everything you need. In fact, the only reason it can't be carried on indefinitely is because there are some food groups that have been ignored, and which should really be included for optimum health.

You may also wish to cut out just a few elements of your diet – including wheat, for example, or perhaps dairy produce, alcohol, caffeine or meat. As long as you stick to the principles of the diet, which is to choose whole, fresh foods rather than those that are processed, refined or containing food additives, it is perfectly possible to make only a few changes. We have cut most of these foods and drinks from *Perfect Detox* because they tend to put pressure on your detox organs and your digestion, and are also most commonly implicated in health problems.

If you are pressed for time, and not up for making broadscale changes, cutting one or two elements out at a time is acceptable. The results may not be as quick or as long-lasting, but if you follow the basics of the diet, and take some liver and kidney support in the form of supplements, therapies or remedies, you will experience positive changes.

The side-effects of detoxing

The end result will undoubtedly be glowing good health, but you should be prepared for some niggling side-effects en route to your destination. *Perfect Detox* is designed to be a gentle healing programme, which won't push you too hard; however, some people may need to slow down a little…

First and foremost, if you experience headaches, nausea, vomiting and general malaise, you may be suffering from the Herxheimer Reaction, which occurs when your body detoxes too rapidly, and toxins are being

Falling off the wagon

Perfect Detox is not a 'diet' as such, and giving in to temptation is not the end of the world. Simply dust yourself off and return to the programme. You may find that eating or drinking foods that you've eliminated from your diet makes you feel light-headed, uncomfortable or even ill! Alcohol and caffeine, in particular, can make you feel pretty rotten after detoxing, as can sugar; that may be enough to put you off overindulgence for the duration and thereafter. You may need to go off-menu for social reasons, and that is acceptable too. In reality, however, it is usually possible to eat whatever is on offer by sticking to vegetables, whole grains, pulses and fish. If any of the foods on the 'no-no' list makes it on to your plate, you can either avoid them, or resolve to get back on the wagon the following day.

If you are struggling to carry on, perhaps because you have experienced some uncomfortable symptoms, try some of the remedies on pages 68–72. Flower essences in particular can be very useful.

released faster than your body can eliminate them. Even though this is a short-term problem, it can put you off continuing. To minimise these effects, make sure you drink plenty of water, get at least a little exercise daily, reduce your intake of herbal supplements, take a sauna or steam bath to help encourage the release of toxins and increase your dosage of psyllium husks and seeds, which will help to clear out your colon. Gentle herbs and their oils, such as chamomile, will help to soothe and calm. You may also wish to consider a massage, which will encourage speedy elimination.

Not everyone experiences such an extreme reaction, but there are other symptoms that can sometimes result at the outset of your detox. These include:

• Headaches, which are particularly common if you regularly drank caffeine or alcohol, or had a bit of a sugar addiction.

- Constipation, which is the result of a change in your diet.
- Fatigue and lethargy, which occurs when your body is kick-started into action, and has to work hard for a few days to get going. Some people call this a 'healing crisis', because it is a good sign that your body has begun to work.
- Aches and pains are often experienced, and are the result of toxins entering the bloodstream. You may also feel nauseous.
- Irritability, which is the result of toxins affecting your brain and nervous system, and an emotional effect of removing foods to which you may have become addicted or dependent.
- Darkly coloured urine, which is a sign of toxins being removed through your urine, and the effect of the various fruit and vegetables you may be eating (or drinking). For example, beets, blueberries and asparagus can all produce some brightly coloured urine. B vitamins also turn your urine very yellow. You'll be aiming for clear urine, rather than dark yellow or brown, so continue to drink lots of water until you reach this point.
- Loose bowels may be the result of the fibre you have added to your diet. It make take some time for this to settle down, but it is a positive sign that your body is clearing out waste. In the short term, cut the psyllium husks from your diet.
- Spots can appear as your skin begins to work its magic and expel toxins, and this is very common.
- Runny nose and other discharges often occur at the outset as your body clears out from every available orifice.

Easing the pain

- Drinking plenty of water is the best advice, and adding a gentle natural diuretic (see pages 64–7) will also ensure that your kidneys are stimulated to eliminate as much waste as possible.
- Eat little and often to keep your moods and blood-sugar levels steady. If your body is used to the highs and lows associated with sugar, refined carbs, caffeine and alcohol, you may feel tired and low as your body adjusts.

- Keep up the fibre. Unless you have wildly uncomfortable diarrhoea, continue to eat as much fibre as you can, which will help to encourage the regular expulsion of toxins.
- Rest as often as you can in the first couple of days, which allows your body the energy to heal and recover. Plenty of sleep will also help.
- Use flower essences and aromatherapy oils to support and soothe (see pages 68–70).
- Remember that discomfort only lasts a few days, and you will feel transformed thereafter. Symptoms are normally related to your toxicity, so if you've been on a few benders and eating poorly, you can expect them to be worse.

Ready to go, but stuck for ideas for putting together the ideal menu plan? *Perfect Detox* has that covered too. Read on!

3 Food and drink

There are no particular foods you absolutely have to eat on the *Perfect Detox* programme, but it's a good idea to focus on some of the detox superfoods, which you'll find listed later in the book. These superfoods have some amazing qualities and therapeutic benefits that will not only enhance your *Perfect Detox*, but encourage optimum health and well-being.

Otherwise, as long as you have a wide variety of fresh, wholesome fruit and vegetables, whole grains, pulses and good-quality protein, you'll be getting everything you need. We talked earlier about the importance of variety, and this is one of the single most important things you can do to achieve a successful detox with long-term effects.

Simply follow the guidelines for each of the detox programmes, and then call upon the detox superfoods listed at the back of the book to create varied, interesting and delicious dishes. To help inspire you, we've come up with suggestions for breakfast, lunch, dinner, snacks and even puddings, as well as some tasty recipes to give you an idea of how foods can be put together. You can mix and match them as you wish, making sure that you don't exceed your intake of dairy produce on the 14- and 30-day programmes, and that you aren't overeating fish or eggs, which should be limited for the duration (see pages 34 and 42). Otherwise, you really can't overeat the other foods on this diet; in fact, the more fruit and vegetables, whole grains and pulses you include in your diet, the better you'll feel! We would recommend that you avoid eating more than two handfuls of nuts each day, as they are high in fat (the good type, but high none the less).

Preparing your food

Any of the detox superfoods (see pages 82–122) can be eaten in unlimited quantities, and served raw or cooked, according to your individual tastes. When shopping for your detox programme, and preparing your meals, you may want to bear the following in mind.

What's a portion?

For the purposes of this programme, a portion will be roughly a handful of any raw food. So, a portion of grapes would probably amount to about eight grapes, while two or three good-sized broccoli spears would also be about right. In reality, however, the size of the portions is not crucial. You will want to have a good bowl or plate of food at every meal, and eat until you feel satisfied. So a big bowl of rice may appear to be well over one portion; however, if you serve it alongside a variety of steamed or raw vegetables, and include some pulses, an egg or a serving of fish, you'll have a perfectly balanced meal that will encourage detoxification and meet your nutritional needs. Try to avoid overeating any one food, apart from brown rice (see page 114).

Go for variety

The more varied your diet, the healthier and more nutritious it is likely to be. Research shows that eating a variety of different brightly coloured fruits and vegetables is the best way to ensure that you are getting the correct balance of antioxidant nutrients, as well as other key compounds your body needs to stay healthy and detox effectively. Five servings of fruits and vegetables a day is often recommended; we suggest you go further and aim for up to ten. It's not as difficult as you may think – throwing a handful of mixed berries into a salad, choosing fruit for pudding, drinking plenty of fresh fruit and vegetable juice, and snacking on raw carrots, celery, cucumber, peppers and other crudités will easily help you meet your target.

The same goes for the other foods you eat. Choosing different grains and pulses will supply you with a multitude of key nutrients, all of which play different roles in the body. Similarly, different types of fish will add other important nutrients to ensure that you get the balance right. So, apart from brown rice, aim to choose different fruits and vegetables, pulses and grains at every meal.

Raw or cooked?

Raw foods contain enzymes that are required by the body to break down other foods. Cooking tends to break down these enzymes, whereas in raw foods they remain intact throughout the chewing process, the stomach acid and, some experts believe, the entire digestive system.

But there is another side to the coin. A Europe-wide study has shown that the body can absorb more of an important substance from cooked vegetables than from raw ones. The research suggests that cooking can improve our absorption of carotenoids, one of the key antioxidants (which is found in carrots, broccoli and spinach) when it comes to protecting health. For example, while the gut could absorb between 3 and 4 per cent of the carotenoids in raw carrots, that could increase by up to five times if the carrots were cooked and mashed.

What's the answer? Try to aim for half raw and half cooked, as we have suggested, and you should get it just about right.

Which cooking method?

The very best way to cook your food is to steam it, which helps to preserve the nutrient content without adding any unnecessary fats. You can steam food in your microwave by adding a little water to the bottom of your cooking bowl and covering it with non-PVC wrap. Stir-fries, where food is cooked quickly in a little hot oil such as vegetable oil, sesame oil or olive oil, can also be effective, but make sure the veggies remain crunchy and that you avoid burning. Alternatively, roast vegetables in the oven in a little olive oil. Avoid frying, which allows foods to absorb a lot of oil.

Eating organic

Organic food is grown or produced under strict regulations – under natural conditions, without the use of chemicals – and an organic food kite mark (such as the Soil Association approval stamp) is notoriously difficult to receive. Organic vegetables are grown without artificial fertilisers or pesticides, in ground that has been tested and declared free of contamination. Nothing labelled organic is irradiated or contains any genetically modified organisms, and choosing organic food means avoiding all of the hundreds of additives or E-numbers regularly found in conventional foods. Many additives are known to cause cancer, hyperactivity, insomnia, birth defects, anxiety, asthma and allergies.

Most importantly, perhaps, organic food is higher in vitamins, minerals and other nutrients. This has been an area of dispute, with some experts claiming that organic food is no better for us nutritionally, but there is now plenty of research to support the fact that organic is better. The Soil Association, the British organisation that campaigns for organic farming, found that organic foods contain more 'secondary metabolites' than conventionally grown plants. Secondary metabolites are substances which form part of plants' immune systems, and which also help to fight cancer in humans. They claim that research from Denmark and Germany shows that '… organic crops also have a measurably higher level of vitamins, and that this can benefit people who eat them. By contrast, intensive farming is devitalising our food.'

Organic produce is also believed to have higher vitamin C levels than non-organic, and organic tomatoes have been found to contain 23 per cent more vitamin A than conventional ones. Vitamins C and A are two of the antioxidants that can help to prevent cancer and heart disease, and, in some cases, reverse it.

Taking this one step further, it can be even more beneficial to eat organic produce grown locally (and therefore seasonally). First, there are clear environmental issues – food flown halfway across the world is responsible for one of the biggest sources of carbon emissions. Second, local produce tends to be far fresher, which preserves its nutrient content (and also the taste!). For example, some studies show that green beans lose up to 60 per cent of their original vitamin C during the first three days of refrigeration after harvesting.

The purpose of a *Perfect Detox* is to eliminate as many toxins as possible while providing your body with the best sources of all the nutrients it needs. For this reason, organic is always your best bet. If you are on a tight budget, don't panic. Purchase as much as you can afford, and focus on the foods that you are likely to eat the most often, such as brown rice, apples or salad, for example. Choosing organic food in season is often cheaper, and will help you to get a good variety of different fruit and vegetables that you may not have considered before.

Breakfast

It's very important to eat breakfast, as it will give you the energy you need to face the day, and also encourage healthy digestion. If you can't stomach a meal, then go for a smoothie or some freshly pressed or squeezed fruit and vegetable juices (see page 156), along with a handful of nuts and an oatcake or two. You might also consider the following:

- Fresh fruit, such as berries, melon and citrus fruit, topped with live yoghurt and a swirl of Manuka honey.
- Porridge soaked overnight in water, with soya milk and Manuka honey, or fresh fruit purée (see page 151).
- Oatmeal topped with dried fruit, raw nuts and a little maple syrup.
- Oatcakes with fresh fruit purée or unsalted, unsweetened nut butter.
- Poached eggs on a bed of wilted spinach.
- Banana oatmeal: oatmeal made with water and topped with natural yoghurt, banana and raisins, and sweetened with honey.
- Eggs scrambled with water, chives, a little live yoghurt and topped with some naturally smoked poached haddock.
- Rye bread with goat's cheese (on the 30-day programme only) and mixed fresh herbs or a mixture of apples, walnuts and dried apricots.
- Smoothies made from fresh or frozen fruit and live yoghurt – if you like them cold and thick, freeze a banana, and pop it into the

liquidiser. Consider fruits you may not associate with smoothies, such as grapefruit or cranberries, which can help to purify. Mango, papaya and mint are lovely together, too. If you are avoiding all dairy on this plan, use unsweetened brown rice milk or organic soya milk instead of yoghurt.

- Vanilla smoothie: blend rice milk, a chopped pear, lychees and a drop of vanilla essence. Sprinkle with finely chopped raw nuts.
- Fresh fruit salad with a dressing made from plain yoghurt, tangerine juice, a drop of pure vanilla essence and cinnamon.
- Apple flaxseed pancakes (see page 125).
- Peanut butter and banana corn quesadillas (see page 125).
- Fruity quinoa (see page 126).
- Maple millet (see page 124).
- Baked apples (see page 124).
- Fruit salad of mango, papaya and melon, topped with sesame seeds and honey.

Lunch

Eating regularly will help to keep your digestive system working efficiently and prevent swings in your blood sugar that could lead to cravings, irritability, headaches and fatigue. Get as many fresh fruits and veggies into your lunch as you can – you can never have too many! All of these lunch ideas can be made easily at home, and most can be put together for a packed lunch. Consider investing in a wide-mouthed thermos flask, which will allow you to take hot meals out and about.

- Baked sweet potato with tzaziki (see page 151) and steamed salmon.
- Brown rice salad, with chopped peppers, braised aubergine and courgettes, and baked cherry tomatoes in a lemon herb dressing (see page 146). Top with lightly toasted sesame and sunflower seeds for extra crunch, fibre, essential fatty acids and a little protein.
- Nettle soup (see page 127) with warmed oatcakes or rye bread.
- Hearty vegetable soup (see page 131) with non-wheat bread.

- A Mediterranean vegetable omelette, with red onion, cherry tomatoes, courgette and peppers; if you are on the 30-day plan, top with goat's cheese or a little feta.
- Vegetable curry with brown rice (see page 129).
- Stuffed bell peppers (see page 128).
- Homemade chickpea or pea hummus (see pages 147, 150), with oatcakes and a green salad bursting with fresh vegetables.
- Fresh Niçoise salad, with grilled tuna, steamed green beans, black olives and any combination of fresh or grilled vegetables, served on a bed of Romaine lettuce with lemon herb dressing (see page 146).
- Greek salad, with Romaine lettuce, cucumbers, black olives, cherry tomatoes, red onion, sliced roasted peppers and chunks of feta (on the 30-day programme only). Replace the feta with pecans for an interesting option, and serve with fresh oregano dressing.
- Ratatouille (see page 128) on brown rice or wheat-free bread.
- Corn or quinoa pasta with steamed vegetables and an easy tomato sauce (see page 152).
- Quinoa salad with roasted vegetables of any description; serve with fresh oregano dressing (see page 147).
- Quinoa salad with almonds, raisins, dried apricot, mango and apple chunks, walnuts and pumpkin seeds, dressed with herb lemon dressing (see page 146).
- Marinated vegetable kebabs (see page 130) served with brown rice and a green salad.
- Crunchy guacamole (see page 148) served with oatcakes and crudités, or in a corn tortilla with red and black beans.
- Corn on the cob drizzled with olive oil and a shake of paprika, with three-bean salad (see page 141).
- Lentil salad with walnuts and goat's cheese (see page 143).

Dinner

A light dinner can help to ensure that you aren't still digesting your food at bedtime; however, it is important to get plenty of fibre, to keep nutrients and toxins moving through your system. If dinner is normally your main meal, try to eat at least five hours before bedtime. You can choose from any of the lunch ideas, and reduce or increase the quantities accordingly. A protein-rich dinner can help to encourage restful sleep, and good-quality whole grains will make sure you don't have a hunger attack mid-evening or during the night!

- Honey-roasted salmon (see page 137) with sweet potato and parsnip mash (see page 139), served with roasted asparagus.
- Tuna skewers (see page 140) with spinach raita (see page 150), brown rice and carrot salad (see page 142).
- Lentil moussaka (see page 136) with green salad.
- Sesame stir-fry with brown rice (see page 138).
- Haddock poached in apricot juice, with warm, fruity quinoa salad (see page 144).
- Chickpea curry with brown rice (see page 133).
- Grilled salmon with watercress salad (see page 144) and beets.
- Grilled salmon or tuna with tzaziki (see page 151), avocado salad and butter bean mash (see page 133).
- Creamy fish pie with pine-nut crust (see page 134)
- Stir-fried tofu with winter vegetables and brown rice (see page 139).
- Fish and lemon tagine with green olives and brown rice (see page 135).
- Corn or quinoa pasta with watercress pesto (see page 152).
- Rye bread topped with fresh salmon and tzaziki (see page 151), accompanied by a green salad.
- Throw as many green herbs together as you can gather, and toss with some rocket, Romaine lettuce and baby leaves; drizzle with lemon juice, a sprinkling of sea salt and some olive oil, and top with lightly toasted pine nuts and pieces of freshly sliced avocado. With some tofu, veggie kebabs or fish, you have a perfect meal.
- A tricolore salad doesn't necessarily involve dairy. Instead, slice fresh tomatoes, ripe avocado and top with chopped basil, lightly toasted pine nuts and thinly sliced black olives. Drizzle with a little balsamic vinegar and olive oil, and use plenty of black pepper.

- Throw cooked brown rice, quinoa, seeds, nuts and cooked lentils into any salad, stew, casserole or soup to give crunch, variety and extra nutrients.

Puddings

There's nothing like something sweet to finish off a meal, and the *Perfect Detox* programme positively encourages you to indulge, as every one of these delicious puddings is guaranteed to add nutrients and fibre to your diet. Any of the breakfast suggestions also makes a good finale for your evening meal, so don't hesitate to experiment.

- Poached pears (see page 154).
- Peach and rhubarb compote with live yoghurt (see page 155).
- Apple and raisin crumble (see page 153).
- Fresh mango and papaya slices, drizzled with honey and sprinkled with mint.
- Pomegranate ice (see page 155).
- Fresh figs with goat's cheese (on the 30-day programme only).
- Baked figs (see page 154).
- Fresh fruit salad with sweet orange dressing (see page 146).

Snacks

Keeping your blood-sugar levels steady will encourage the detoxification process and also provide you with the energy you need to heal. What's more, snacking offers an opportunity to increase your intake of key detox foods (see pages 82–122), and all of them make great options for between meals.

- Plain popcorn – air-popped, or popped with a little olive oil.
- Fresh fruit.
- Dried unsulphured fruit.

- Oatcakes or unsalted rice cakes with fresh fruit purée (see page 151), hummus (see page 147), crunchy guacamole (see page 148) or raw nut butters.
- Raw seeds and nuts.
- Crudités with dip (see pages 148–9 for ideas).
- Small portions of any of the meal ideas.
- Plain yoghurt with fresh fruit and nuts.

Stuck for inspiration?

If cooking isn't your forte, or you haven't come across some of these super detox foods before, we've got a fantastic compendium of delicious, nutritious detox recipes at the back of the book (see pages 123–57). Don't be afraid to create unusual food combinations – sometimes the most original, tasty meals come straight from your imagination!

Food is just one part of a successful detox. There is a multitude of herbs, oils, remedies, supplements, therapies and other treatments that are specially designed to encourage detoxification and look after the organs involved. While changing your diet and lifestyle will undoubtedly have a dramatic impact on your overall health, there is also additional help at hand to encourage the process and get healing under way. In the next chapter you'll find everything you need to make your *Perfect Detox* a success.

4 Detox aids

Everyone needs a little help from time to time, and there is a wealth of tried-and-tested remedies and treatments to encourage the detoxification process, and support your liver, kidneys and other organs in the process. All of these are readily available at good health-food shops, larger pharmacies, and on the internet. Let's look at some of the best that are on offer.

Supplements

There are many that help to encourage the process of detoxification, while supporting the action of the main detox organs, such as the skin, liver and kidneys as well as the bowel. By adding these to your diet, or getting them in the form of food (see pages 82–122 for details of foods that are high in these detox superstars), you can increase the rate at which toxins are removed from the body, as well as improve your health on all levels. What's more, you'll be less likely to suffer from side-effects during the detox itself.

Multi-vitamins and minerals

Even the healthiest diet may not contain the key nutrients that our bodies need to function at optimum level. In some cases this is because foods travel long distances before they reach our supermarket shelves, thereby diminishing their nutrient content; many of our foods are processed, too, which compromises them even further. Several studies have found that food simply isn't as nutritious as it once was, perhaps because the soil from which plants (and the animals who feed on them) get their own vitamins and minerals has been exhausted of its nutrients by intensive farming methods. Whatever the cause, you'll do well to add a multi-vitamin and mineral to your diet while undertaking the detox, and to continue to do so for at least three months afterwards to ensure that your body has what it needs to perform efficiently.

The liver requires certain nutrients for detox. Increasing the flow of bile is important because bile carries stored fat-soluble toxins away from the liver to be excreted in the stools. In particular, antioxidants – like vitamins A, E and in particular C (which aids the detoxification process in several ways, especially by recycling other antioxidants such as glutathione and vitamin E), as well as the minerals zinc and selenium – are essential for detoxification. When our antioxidant levels are low, energy is not available and detoxification cannot take place in a normal fashion. Therefore, toxins accumulate or are stored until they can be processed. A good multi-vitamin and mineral tablet will supply antioxidants, as well as other nutrients that are critical to the detoxification process.

These include:

- **Magnesium,** which is a crucial factor in the natural self-cleansing and detoxification responses of the body. It stimulates the sodium-potassium pump on the cell wall and this initiates the cleansing process. It also protects the cells from heavy metals and other toxins, and is involved in both phases of liver detoxification.
- **Potassium**, which is involved in almost every body process, and which tends to be depleted when we have inadequate diets, crash diet or take diuretics (even natural ones). Potassium cleanses and restores.
- **Folic acid**, which supports the healthy metabolism of fat in the liver, and encourages bile flow. It also promotes balanced detoxification.
- **Zinc**, which encourages most of the enzyme reactions between minerals and is used in phase I detoxification. Zinc also improves liver function in general.

- **Selenium**, which aids in the production of the antioxidant enzyme glutathione, which detoxifies your body (see page 61). Selenium also protects the liver from alcoholic cirrhosis (and therefore from the damaging toxins it contains).
- **Molybdenum**, which detoxifies alcohol, helps to remove nitrogen waste from the body by the formation of uric acid (a powerful antioxidant), detoxifies sulphites (food preservatives), and functions as a co-factor of various enzymes involved in the detoxification process.
- **Beta-carotene**, the precursor to vitamin A, is a powerful antioxidant that protects the liver from damage and helps support detoxification mechanisms.
- **Biotin**. Liver cells that lack biotin will be deprived of the energy they need to detoxify chemicals and drugs. Deficiency of this vitamin is rare but it can cause hair loss, dry, flaky skin, rashes and fatigue. Those with a poor diet, alcoholism or long-term antibiotic use are at risk of deficiency.
- **B-complex vitamins**, which are synergistic, meaning they work together. B vitamins are among the first vitamins to be depleted under stress when toxins are present. It's important to replenish the B-complex vitamins during a detox programme. They also help to balance hormones and lift energy during the detoxification process, and nourish the nervous system.
- **Choline** is from the B family of vitamins, but it is mentioned separately here because of its crucial importance to the detox process. It offers powerful support for the kidneys and reduces inflammation. It has also been used successfully for the treatment of fatty liver disease and other forms of liver damage, encouraging regeneration and the detoxification process.

Digestive enzymes

These are important not only for digestion, but also for detoxification. They are best obtained from fresh, raw fruit and vegetables (see some of the detox superfoods listed later in the book), but digestive enzymes can also be taken as supplements, particularly if your diet has been very poor over the years.

Enzymes will help to cleanse the bowel, because they help to break down foods for digestion and absorption, making them more liquid and able to be transported more easily and quickly through the digestive system – thus removing and eliminating toxins before they can cause trouble. What's more, by ensuring that food is properly digested, and its nutrients absorbed and assimilated by your body, your liver will get the nutrients it needs to produce its own enzymes. Enzymes are necessary to break down all types of foods, and thus they provide support to your liver both during detoxification and afterwards.

Always supplement with an enzyme that has both upper (such as, papain, HCL, etc.) and lower (such as amalyse, lactase, etc.) digestive enzymes. Most digestive enzymes have lower (pancreatic) enzymes from plant sources but not the upper stomach enzymes. Take them between meals, rather than before or during, to encourage your body to produce and create its own.

SAMe

There are certain natural compounds, found in foods or manufactured by your body, that are strongly 'lipotropic' – meaning they remove fat from your liver and allow it to function normally again. One such substance is a derivative of the amino acid methionine, called s-adenosyl methionine (or SAMe). It is normally produced in your liver from methionine, folic acid and vitamin B12. However, it stops being produced in sufficient quantities if your liver is clogged up with fat.

SAMe protects your liver from the effects of harmful chemicals, which must pass through your liver to be detoxified. It also promotes the flow of bile, which is essential for the digestion of fats and for the absorption of the fat-soluble vitamins A, D, E and K. Taking supplements of SAMe has been found to help restore normal liver function, even in people with more serious liver diseases, such as cirrhosis.

Probiotics

These healthy bacteria are introduced to the gut to ensure that it is balanced and working at optimum level. They are pretty much essential during any detox diet, not only because a thorough cleanse tends to wipe out your healthy bacteria population alongside the toxins, but also because unhealthy guts are usually overpopulated by unhealthy strains of bacteria, which need to be balanced by the introduction of healthy strains such as acidophilus. Probiotics encourage healing of the gut, as well as supporting a healthy immune system. The health of the gut has a substantial impact on the health of the liver, as everything absorbed from the intestines passes through the liver in order for harmful substances to be detoxified before the rest of the body is exposed to them.

Prebiotics are non-digestible foods that encourage good bacteria to grow and flourish. They help to restore the balance in your gut, and are found in certain types of fibre, including inulin.

Glutathione

Glutathione is a powerful antioxidant composed of the amino acids cysteine, glutamine and glycine, and is concentrated in the liver although it carries out its work throughout the body. This important enzyme is involved in protecting cells from environmental toxins, drugs and alcohol, as well as normal toxins produced by the body in the process of metabolism. It is also involved in a healthy immune system. Glutathione has a synergistic effect with other antioxidants to protect the body against free radicals, and it attaches itself to toxic chemicals and drugs in the liver and renders them into a state suitable for elimination from the body.

Essential fatty acids (EFAs)

As their name suggests, these are essential oils – fats, in fact – and your body needs them! Essential fatty acids, which come from foods, are converted into substances that keep the blood thin, lower blood pressure, decrease inflammation, improve the function of the nervous and immune systems, help insulin to work, affect vision, co-ordination and mood, encourage healthy metabolism and maintain the balance of water in our bodies. These essential fats are a vital component of every human cell and the body also needs them to insulate nerve cells, keep the skin and arteries supple and to keep warm. Best of all, EFAs encourage healthy liver and kidney function (in particular, supporting liver regeneration), and play a role in balancing hormones, which take pressure off the liver.

Sadly, our diets are usually deficient in these key fats, which are also known as the 'omega' oils – 3, 6 and 9. Good vegetarian sources include green plants, nuts and seeds; other key sources are freshwater fish and their oils. Vegetarian sources have one advantage over fish oils, in that they are rich sources of vitamin E, which is required to keep our arteries healthy and our skin looking youthful. Many of us do not get enough in our diets which is why a supplement is advisable, not only while detoxing, but also on a daily basis. Go for flaxseed and/or fish oils, and take as directed. The former is not absorbed quite as efficiently as the latter, but makes a great addition to your detox diet, and is extremely rich in the antioxidant vitamin E.

Herbal remedies

Herbs can be powerful healers, and play a multitude of roles in the body. However, although they are natural, they must be used in moderation and according to the instructions on any packaging. More doesn't mean better, even if the herbs you choose seem to be making a dramatic difference to your health.

Herbs come in many forms, including capsules, tisanes (much like a teabag or dried, loose tea) and tinctures (herbs are decocted or infused, and then suspended in water and alcohol). You may find tinctures the easiest to manage, and they can be added to food or drink to disguise their flavour. The other way to include herbs in your diet is, of course, to eat them fresh, in salads or as flavourings for food.

In our A–Z of detox superfoods (see pages 82–122), we look at some of the herbs that are widely used in cooking. Below you'll find still others that can be added to your diet to improve your health and detoxification process even further.

Artichoke extract

On page 84 we discuss the benefits of artichokes themselves. Artichoke extract is taken from the leaves, and a number of studies have found that it enhances the detoxification process of the liver and protects it from the toxic by-products of this process. It also acts as a choleretic, transporting toxins from the liver in the form of bile. Bile is essential for digesting fats, helping to soften stools and keeping the small intestine free of parasites. By encouraging its production, you will effectively speed up the process of detoxification, almost instantly. It also encourages the health of the gall bladder.

In addition, artichoke extract contains antioxidant flavonoids (such as luteolin and apigenin) that have been shown to support a healthy circulatory system, which includes your heart.

Ashwaganda

This herb, also known as 'winter cherry', has had a long and successful history of use in traditional Indian medicine, known as Ayurveda. Ashwaganda helps the body adapt to stress, but it also rebuilds the nervous system without stimulating it, which makes it an effective balancer for the entire body. It may help to encourage a healthy immune system, and research has found that it helps produce restful sleep, which can encourage healing on all levels.

Ashwaganda is rich in phytochemicals such as withananine, choline, trapino and alkaloids, which support the detoxification process and help to mop up toxins. It also helps to balance hormones, which takes pressure off the liver itself. And it has strong anti-inflammatory properties as well.

Buchu

Buchu preparations, which are taken from the leaves of this South African shrub, have a long history of use in traditional herbal medicine as a urinary tract disinfectant and diuretic, which encourages healthy elimination and the health of the kidneys. It was long used by the Hottentot tribe as a cleanser and vitality tonic, and as a mild diuretic; it keeps the toxins flowing! Use it daily for a month, even if you choose a shorter detox programme, to encourage deep-level cleansing.

Cleavers

Cleavers is a wonderful detox herb, working to cleanse the blood and lymph, as well as supporting the liver and kidneys. It is a mild diuretic, which affects the lymphatic system, preventing congestion and swollen lymph nodes (glands). This action also encourages the elimination of waste, and promotes lymphatic drainage of toxins through the urinary system. Its bitter properties stimulate liver function, and enhance the digestion and absorption of a multitude of nutrients.

Dandelion root

Both dandelion roots and leaves are used to encourage and support detoxification and the liver itself (see also page 96). Dandelion acts as a mild diuretic, but also contains potassium, which ensures that imbalances do not occur (see page 58). The roots act as a blood purifier that helps both the kidneys and the liver to remove toxins and poisons from the blood, and they have also been used for centuries to treat jaundice. Dandelion acts as a mild laxative and improves appetite and digestion. German research has shown that dandelion root is a mild bitter, which acts to increase bile production and bile flow in the liver. This makes it useful for people with sluggish liver function due to alcohol abuse or poor diet. It is restorative to the liver and helps reduce the risk of developing gallstones (although it shouldn't be used if you do have them).

Juniper berries

Juniper berries may strengthen and detoxify the kidneys, bladder and urinary tract. While juniper is excellent for cleansing purposes – its diuretic action increases the filtration rate of the kidneys – long-term use is not recommended as it can overtax the kidneys, where it causes local irritation. The frequent use of juniper may be harmful and should be avoided by those suffering from kidney disease or diabetes, and also by pregnant women or those who are breastfeeding. It is also not recommended for use by people with a kidney infection.

Milk thistle

This herb is the most essential of all detox herbs, and plays a powerful role in protecting the liver. Milk thistle has been used to treat inflammation of the liver, hepatitis, mushroom and chemical poisoning, as well as liver damage from alcohol abuse or long-term use of certain medications. And there is plenty of research to back this up.

German scientists began investigating the properties of milk thistle some years ago, and found a concentrated group of flavonoids, known as silymarin. Flavonoids are key antioxidants that neutralise free radicals in the bloodstream, which harm cells and accelerate the process of ageing. Silymarin flavonoids were found to be 'antihepatoxic', which means that they act directly on the liver to protect it from toxins and other poisons.

They work on two levels, first by binding to the membranes of liver cells to produce a protective shield, which prevents toxins from penetrating the cell walls. Second, they stimulate, speeding up the production of healthy enzymes and proteins, to encourage healing and regeneration when toxins do make it to the cells.

Milk thistle also increases the activity of glutathione, the body's own antioxidant, which scavenges free radicals, detoxifies heavy metals, helps ferry amino acids into the cells, helps in bile production, protects the liver, supports kidney function – and much more.

Psyllium husks and seeds

This fibre-rich herb acts as a gentle natural laxative and it thus cleanses the digestive tract and prevents the build-up of hardened material. The gel that forms when psyllium is taken (with plenty of water) attracts and absorbs toxins as it passes through the bowels, and addresses those that may be tucked away in colon pockets. What's more, it slows down the transit of food in the digestive system, encouraging better assimilation and helping to balance blood-sugar levels. And because the liver dumps into the bowels, via the gall bladder, keeping the bowels clean and moving is of major importance to regular detoxification.

Red clover

Red clover is a mild diuretic, known as a 'blood cleanser', and has been studied for its ability to keep harmful toxins from the lymphatic system, which runs parallel to the circulatory system and is responsible for filtering cellular waste. It's also a potent liver purifier, and stimulates bile production, which is essential for good digestion. Red clover encourages healthy skin, which makes elimination through the sweat glands more efficient. Finally, it's a potent hormone stabiliser, which can help to take pressure off the liver.

Schizandra

A number of studies have found that schizandra, a woody vine native to China and Japan, protects the liver from toxic build-up. It can also boost the immune system by helping the liver to eliminate toxins that have built up over time. Other studies have found that it protects against the effects of alcohol, and encourages the regeneration of the liver. It contains more than 30 lignins (chemicals in plants known as phyto-estrogens), which are beneficial to the liver and enhance its regenerative properties, and it is also known to increase metabolism, stimulating the production of enzymes in the liver and in the digestive system, which contributes to detoxification.

Slippery elm

This soothing herb is often included in detox blends. It acts as a 'demul-cent', meaning that it forms a soothing film over mucous membranes, encouraging healing and intestinal balance, improving digestion and gently cleansing. It helps to soften the stool, which can discourage the build-up of hardened intestinal plaque or waste deposits, and encour-ages healthy elimination. It is a natural anti-inflammatory, which works on all mucous membranes in the body including the lungs, thereby encouraging healthy breathing, bringing oxygen to the blood and through that to all the cells in the body.

Uva ursi

Uva ursi is a herb traditionally used to help fight bacteria in the urinary tract and cleanse it. It has antiseptic qualities, which help to tone and support the urinary tract and kidney function. The quercetin (see under 'Onions', page 108) contained in uva ursi acts to protect the capillaries that make up the delicate kidney filtering system. It also helps to stabilise blood-sugar levels, which is crucial during a detox, and to provide support for the pancreas and liver during cleansing.

Yarrow

Yarrow, a flowering plant, has been shown to have anti-inflammatory properties, in particular acting on the urinary tract. It has also been shown in a few different studies to help regulate liver function. Yarrow acts as a blood cleanser, and encourages the pores to open, thereby elim-inating waste and relieving the kidneys. It has been traditionally used to tone the mucus membranes in the stomach and bowel, encouraging healthy digestion and good bacteria or 'gut flora'.

Essential oils

Aromatherapy oils use the 'life force' of plants for therapeutic purposes, and can be added to your bath (5 drops is about right), used in massage (3–4 drops in a carrier oil, such as grapeseed, olive or sweet almond, for example), or spritzed in your environment.

There are a number of oils that specifically support or encourage the detoxification process. They can be used together to create a combination that will address your individual needs. For example, for your liver and lymphatic system, blend a drop each of geranium, rosemary, Roman chamomile, fennel, carrot, German chamomile, helichrysum and blue tansy. This combination cleanses the liver and the lymphatic system of high levels of toxins. Use a few drops of this mix, as required. Other specific oils include:

- **Juniper** is a potent detoxifying oil, with astringent and antiseptic qualities. It encourages healthy circulation which will speed up elimination. It also acts as a diuretic to increase the expulsion of toxins and waste, as well as encouraging metabolism. It's powerful, so use only a couple of drops.
- **Fennel** encourages digestion, and helps to prevent water retention by working as a diuretic. It acts as an antiseptic to the urinary tract and kidneys, and as a general tonic, increasing circulation to remove waste and toxins from the bloodstream.
- **Lemon** stimulates white blood cells, and has detoxifying and regeneration properties that are beneficial to the liver and kidneys. It can be harsh on sensitive skin, so use only one drop, well diluted in a carrier oil.
- **Grapefruit** is antiviral, antiseptic and a diuretic, and works specifically on the digestion and skin. It is believed to stimulate bile production in the liver, and has been used to help withdrawal symptoms in detox clinics.
- **Patchouli** is a powerful diuretic, which encourages healthy elimination, flushing toxins through the kidneys. It is an

adaptogenic, which means that it provides energy when required, but also relaxes during periods of stress, working on the adrenal glands to support balance.

- **Helichrysum** is excellent for detoxing drugs and alcohol. It stimulates the liver cells, thins mucous secretions and acts as an antioxidant.
- **Geranium** is a diuretic oil, and stimulates both the liver and kidneys. It also works directly on the lymphatic system, improving immunity, and it boosts circulation, providing oxygenated blood to organs and helping with elimination.
- **Black pepper** works directly on the colon, encouraging healthy elimination and digestion. It stimulates the circulation and supports liver function. It's another powerful oil, so only a drop in a carrier oil or in the bath will do the trick.

Detoxification baths

Salt baths, or baths using any of the essential oils that encourage detoxification, can be a useful addition to your detox programme, encouraging elimination of toxins through the skin. Hot water draws toxins out of the body to the skin's surface, and while the water cools it pulls toxins from the skin. Epsom salts encourage this process of detoxification by causing you to sweat. Other salts – all highly alkaline and cleansing – that can be used in baths include sea salt, bicarbonate of soda, clay and Dead Sea salts.

To make your own detox bath, try adding two good handfuls of Epsom salts (or the equivalent of bicarbonate of soda or sea salt) to a hot bath. Soak for 15–20 minutes, and then scrub your skin gently with a loofah or organic flannel. The water will turn murky in colour, which is a sign that toxins are being drawn out. Repeat once a week during your detox, and then once a month thereafter for maintenance.

Flower essences

Flower essences harness the vibration or 'energy' of a flower's petals or leaves, and work to address negative emotions that can be the cause of imbalance and illness. Many people find them useful during the process of detoxification, as they provide support and help to purify on a number of different levels. Why not try:

- **Purifying Essence**, an Australian Bush Flower Essence, which combines the following flower essences: bush iris, bottlebrush, dagger hakea, dog rose and wild potato bush. The aim is to release and clear emotional waste and to encourage 'spring-cleaning'.
- **Yarrow flower** essence detoxes the body and mind, and strengthens.
- Mountain devil is good for detoxification and deep cleansing, particularly if you are feeling angry and irritable.
- **Rescue Remedy**, a Bach Flower Remedy, helps with the side-effects of detox (see pages 43–6) and can help to relieve irritability, headaches and concentration problems.
- **Crab apple**, another Bach remedy, is cleansing, and particularly good if you feel 'unclean' on an emotional or physical level.
- **Peruvian Amazon Courage Orchid**, which is one of the Rainforest flower essences, can help with your spirit of conviction, and give you courage to reach your goals.

Homeopathic remedies

Homeopathy is a system of treating ill-health on all levels (both emotional and physical) with gentle remedies that act to stimulate our bodies' own healing mechanisms. In much the same way as a radio signal, this affects the energy of our bodies with remedies that have their own 'healing energy', addressing symptoms by providing minute doses of substances that would, in large doses, actually *cause* illness. They work by kick-starting the body to heal itself as it responds to the substance at hand. As a tool for detox, they can be invaluable; however, you may wish to see a registered homeopath who can choose remedies that are most suitable for you and your individual constitution.

Remedies can be taken for up to ten days, should be taken between meals and without coffee or mint (including toothpaste), which can nullify their impact. So, steer well away from snacks, hot drinks or brushing your teeth (about 25 minutes either side is fine). Take the potency suggested. If you wish, you can dilute them in water and sip as required throughout the day. You'll see a number next to the remedy, which represents the 'dilution'. Look out for 6 or 30, which are the best 'dilutions' for treating physical health.

- **Nux vomica** 6 or 30 is a great detoxifier via the digestive system, and it is ideal for anyone who has overdone it – too much alcohol, smoking, fatty or spicy foods, etc. It is highly effective for cleansing toxins from the breakdown of drugs and alcohol, as well as from a poor diet. It reaches the urinary tract organs by repairing damage done by toxin elimination and provides organic support during a detoxification programme.
- **Bryonia** 6 or 30 provides overall digestive support, and is a wonderful liver remedy, providing support and stimulating function.
- **Berberis** 6 or 30 stimulates the kidneys and gall bladder, and is ideal if your excretory organs (liver, kidneys and skin) have been overloaded. It supports the health of the urinary tract.
- **Lycopodium** 6 or 30 supports the lymphatic system and it is a well-known remedy for digestive complaints, especially indigestion, vomiting and bloating, flatulence and constipation. It supports the healthy action of the kidneys, liver and gall bladder, and can help with water retention, encouraging healthy elimination.
- **Nat sulph** 6 or 30 helps to prevent water retention, and encourages the health of the liver, while offering support. It is a good remedy for constipation, stimulating healthy elimination.
- **Colocynthis** 6 or 30 stimulates the natural process of detoxification, both internally and externally.

- **Calc phos** 6 or 30 is a remedy to encourage healthy digestion, and is ideal for a sluggish circulation. It's also an excellent supportive remedy for convalescing.
- **Nat phos** 6 or 30 boosts metabolism and healthy elimination.
- **Kali sulph** 6 or 30 supports the natural detoxification process in the body and strengthens liver functions. It's ideal for putrid discharges (mucus or pus, for example), and for a good-clear out.
- **Sulphur** 6 or 30 is another very good clear-out remedy, and is particularly indicated for helping to excrete heavy metals.

Skin detoxification

Although detoxification works from the inside out, it is important to keep your 'outsides' clean as well, in order to ensure that the process is efficient. The skin is the largest organ in the body, and removes toxins from the body via sweat (perspiration), through the sweat glands. Heavy metals, among other toxins, are excreted through the skin's pores. Therefore it is important to stimulate this process and to encourage the health of your skin, so that it can do its job more effectively. There is a variety of methods you can try.

Saunas and steam rooms

These promote sweating and are therefore ideal for releasing toxins. Make sure you drink plenty of water to replace that which is lost; in fact, topping yourself up in advance of a trip to the sauna or steam room can encourage the 'flushing' action.

Steam and heat treatments help to unblock the pores, which can become clogged with skin products and a build-up of fat-soluble toxins. Some experts recommend that you undertake 15 minutes of aerobic exercise (see pages 34–6) before the treatment to encourage the circulation, which helps to release toxins from fat cells into the bloodstream where they can be efficiently removed.

Dry skin brushing

Brushing the skin works to remove dead skin and oils from the surface of the skin and the pores, enabling them to 'breathe' properly and release waste products. Furthermore, when you brush the skin, you encourage circulation and the action of the lymphatic system, which works to eliminate toxins more speedily. Use a loofah or specially designed dry skin brush. Start at the soles of the feet and work your way up your legs, your front and your back, brushing as vigorously as you feel able. Then do your hands and up your arms. When doing your chest and upper back, focus the brush strokes towards your heart.

Clean skin

Ensuring that your pores are clean and open, not blocked by dirt, oil, make-up and skincare products is extremely important. And that doesn't mean just your face! Detoxification takes place all over your body, and your skin should be carefully cleaned and nourished to keep it moist, supple and 'breathing'. You need to bathe regularly with warm water and natural substances that will work to remove anything clogging your pores.

Natural skincare products

Both for the duration of the detox, and beyond, it makes sense to use natural products on your skin as often as possible. Why? Because the majority of skincare products contain chemicals that can not only increase your toxic load, but also choke your pores. Products that contain healthy, natural ingredients not only encourage the health of your skin, but your whole body as well. What's more, they can actively promote good health through a variety of holistic therapeutic benefits. Consider the following:

- Try using gentle, vegetable-based soaps with essential fatty acids, essential oils and nourishing oils.

- Tone your facial skin with rose or orange blossom water, both of which are cleansing, astringent, moisture-retaining, stimulating and soothing; better still, they stimulate the growth of new, healthy skin cells and protect the skin.
- Moisturise with natural oils such as rose oil, rosehip seed oil or products based on frankincense, all of which work beneath the surface of the skin to act on cell membranes, supporting their immune reaction and initiating their regeneration. Rosehip seed oil, in particular, is an excellent source of topical trans-retinoic acid (vitamin A) in a natural and safe form, which supports the cycle that is responsible for the natural regeneration of skin cells, increasing the number of renewed cells. Natural oils do not seal the skin like many modern-day moisturisers, but allow it to breathe while also providing wonderful hydration.
- Use natural deodorants that are paraben-free and do not contain aluminium. Mineral salts are a good basis for natural deodorants and there are also herbal deodorants, such as those containing tea tree oil, which work to attack the bacteria causing odour. Remember that antiperspirants prevent sweat from forming, which also discourages a very essential part of the detoxification process.
- Use essential oils that encourage detoxification – and soften and nourish the skin – in baths and in place of your usual skincare products (see page 68).
- Look for natural, organic make-up, which will not contain chemicals that provide more work for your body and which will also encourage the health of your skin.

Nourishing the skin

It is equally important that you give your skin the nutrients it needs to stay supple and healthy, allowing it to detoxify at optimum level. Apart from drinking plenty of fresh water throughout the day, cutting out smoking and drinking too much alcohol, keeping your skin protected from excessive sunlight and eating a variety of fresh whole foods, you can consider:

- **MSM** (methylsulphonylmethane), a naturally occurring form of organic sulphur found in all living organisms. Research suggests that sufficient MSM in the body may be critical to both normal function and structure, and as levels in the body tend to drop as we become older, it's even more important to ensure that you have plenty in your diet. You'll find it in milk, meat, fish and most fruits, vegetables and grains.

- **Pine Bark Extract** (Pycnogenol). Certain vitamins and minerals can be called nutritional cosmetics, such is their beneficial impact on the health and vitality of skin, hair and nails. One of the most popular, researched and effective nutritional cosmetics is pine bark extract (the patented form is called Pycnogenol). This is a naturally occurring complex of several antioxidant nutrients, including compounds known as bioflavonoids, fruit acids and proantho-cyanidins (OPCs). OPCs effectively protect collagen structures in several ways. They reinforce the collagen matrix of connective tissue, protect against free-radical damage, and inhibit collagen damage caused by inflammation, infection and the ageing process.

- **Beta-carotene** is a carotenoid, a naturally occurring pigment and potent antioxidant found in red, yellow and orange fruits and vegetables. It is a precursor to vitamin A, which is essential for healthy skin. Prolonged vitamin A deficiency results in a number of symptoms including increased rate of infection and a condition called follicular hyperkeratosis (the build-up of cellular debris in the hair follicles, giving the skin a goose-bump appearance – often found on the backs of the upper arms). Beta-carotene also appears to act as a natural pre-tanning aid and has protective effects against UV damage.

- **Essential Fatty Acids** (EFAs). Good fats, or EFAs, offer numerous health and anti-ageing benefits. Our obsession with fat-free diets has left many people with chronic deficiencies in essential fatty acids, leading to various symptoms including dry, flaky skin, eczema, excessive wrinkling, brittle nails and dry, flyaway or splitting hair. Some of the best sources for the skin include flaxseed oil, hempseed oil, avocado oil, evening primrose oil and pumpkin seed oil.

Detox foot patches

These are incredibly satisfying detox aids, as it is possible to witness just what comes out of your body! They work by drawing out toxins from your feet while you sleep. They are pressed on to the centre of the sole of the foot, and left there for the night. In the morning, these tea-bag shaped patches are normally discoloured and smelly. Regular use is said to keep the body free of excess toxins, including heavy metals. There are a number of foot patches now on the market and, depending on the theory behind each, they are formulated from different ingredients. Whether they are effective in the short or long term is open to debate; however, many people swear by them.

Detox therapies

If you are willing to spend a little money to encourage the process of detoxification, and experience other therapeutic benefits as well, you may want to consider some of the therapies that are known to be helpful. Let's look at some of what's on offer.

Massage

Massage works on several levels, using a variety of different techniques to improve circulation, thereby increasing the flow of toxins from the tissues, providing oxygenated blood to key organs, and encouraging a 'flush'. It helps to cleanse muscle acids, joints, nerves and the endocrine (hormone) system by stimulating the circulatory system and the lymphatic system (which is effectively the body's 'sewage' system).

Deep-tissue techniques remove waste in the muscle tissue, which increases circulation and removes blockages throughout the body that may be preventing healthy elimination. What's more, it can be useful to relax and ease some of the side-effects of detoxification (see pages 43–5).

Manual lymphatic drainage is a form of massage that stimulates the lymphatic system with gentle massaging strokes. The light, rhythmical massage encourages the lymphatic system to eliminate metabolic waste products, excess fluid and bacteria. The effects are numerous and include general benefits to the nervous and muscular systems. MLD is a great addition to other detox measures, as it encourages fluid flow in the connective tissues.

Colonic irrigation

Colonic irrigation, or colonic hydrotherapy, is a therapy designed to remove waste and toxins from the bowel, including impacted faeces, mucus plaque, dead tissue and worms or other parasites. During the procedure, you will lie on your side while warm water is passed into your bowel through a tube that is inserted into your rectum (back passage). This water circulates through your colon in order to encourage your bowel to empty itself. Waste products are then passed out of your body through the tube.

After about ten minutes, you turn on to your back and the therapist gently massages your abdomen to encourage the process. When all of the waste has been removed, you will be offered probiotics (see page 61), to recolonise your gut with healthy bacteria. The aim of colonic irrigation is to improve digestion and elimination, as well as the assimilation of nutrients.

Coffee enemas

Enemas are commonly used in much the same way as colonic irrigation, to flush out toxins and impacted faeces. Enemas involve the introduction of water (usually salty water) into the colon through the rectum. Coffee enemas work a little differently. Some of the many chemicals in coffee – notably caffeine, theophylline and theobromine – combine to stimulate the relaxation of smooth muscles causing dilatation of blood vessels and bile ducts. The enzymes in coffee, known as palmitates, help the liver carry away the toxins in bile acid. The coffee is absorbed and then taken up to the liver. With the bile ducts dilated, bile carries toxins away to the gastrointestinal tract. Simultaneously, the lower colon is flooded, causing it to be evacuated, carrying toxins and bile from the body.

You can visit a therapist to have this treatment undertaken, or you may wish to purchase a kit to do it yourself at home. There are, however, a number of potential side-effects, and people with the following health conditions should not consider it: diverticular disease, ulcerative colitis, Crohn's disease, severe haemorrhoids, blood vessel disease, congestive heart failure, heart disease, severe anaemia, abdominal hernia, gastrointestinal cancer, recent colon surgery and intestinal tumours.

Chelation therapy

The concept of chelation is based on the observation that when an amino acid complex called EDTA (ethylene-diamine-tetra-acetic acid) comes in contact with certain metals and other substances such as lead, iron, copper, calcium, magnesium, zinc, plutonium and manganese, it grabs and removes them.

Chelation therapy is most often given intravenously, either as a short injection or over a period of two to four hours. A typical treatment cycle may include 20 injections or infusions spread over ten to 12 weeks. Chelation therapy can also be given by mouth.

This therapy is frowned upon in some quarters; however, a lot of people swear by it and experience instant effects, such as a reduction in headaches, fatigue, muscle pain, plaque in the cardiovascular system and digestive problems. There are, however, some side-effects, including possible damage to the kidneys. If you are considering this therapy, make sure you choose a reputable, registered and experienced practitioner, who can explain all the pros and cons of treatment.

Cupping

Cupping is a traditional healing technique that promotes circulation and detoxification by stimulating the skin with the application of suction cups – sometimes heated. It has been a popular Western healing tradition since Hippocrates, and the same techniques are used in Chinese and Ayurvedic medicine.

Cupping is helpful for relief from muscle spasms and back pain, as well as arthritic and rheumatic problems. While stimulating the skin and underlying muscles, it promotes the release of toxins that have accumulated in the area and increases circulation of blood and lymph vessels.

Cupping also stimulates the organ-related reflex zones in the skin to further improve the function of inner organs, including the stomach, liver, kidneys and intestines.

There do not appear to be any adverse side-effects to this therapy, and many people find it enormously relaxing. It may be used alongside other therapies, such as acupuncture and some forms of massage.

Relaxation

One of the most important things you can do while detoxing is to undertake some form of relaxation, whether you choose a specific therapy or discipline such as massage, yoga or even acupuncture, aromatherapy or reflexology, or do your own techniques at home. Relaxation helps to encourage the process of detoxification by balancing your system, removing blockages and muscle spasms that may cause energy to stagnate and prevent the effective flow of lymph, which is necessary for healthy excretion of toxins.

Whole-body relaxation

- Find a comfortable position, either on the floor or in a chair. Dim the lighting. Take three deep breaths, breathing right down into your stomach. Breathe in relaxation through the nose, and breathe out all your tension through the mouth.
- Bring your awareness to your right foot. Visualise your big toe, and relax it. Do the same with each right toe in turn – slowly and gently. Continue up your right leg, visualising each part then relaxing it to let the tension go. Do this slowly and purposefully. Don't hurry. Visualise the sole of your right foot, then the top of the foot, the

ankle, shin, calf, knee, front of the thigh, back of the thigh and right buttock. The whole right leg is warm and relaxed. Repeat with your left foot and leg. Slowly.

· Visualise and consciously relax both buttocks. Then, slowly, your lower back, mid-back, space between the shoulder blades, shoulders, neck, scalp, forehead, space between the eyebrows, eyebrows, eyes, eyelids, nose and nostrils, mouth, tongue, jaw, cheeks, chin and head. Your neck, shoulders, face and head are now fully relaxed and warm.

· Slowly move on to visualise and consciously relax your chest, upper abdomen, lower abdomen and pelvis. Now visualise and try to consciously relax all your internal organs – your heart, spleen, liver, kidneys, and so on.

· Bring your awareness to your right arm. Relax the fingers, palm of the hand, wrist, forearm, elbow, upper arm and shoulder. Your whole right arm is relaxed and warm. Repeat on your left arm.

· Your whole body is relaxed and warm. Enjoy the sense of peace. Imagine all your internal organs functioning perfectly, removing toxins from your blood and tissues. You feel cleaner, lighter, healthier.

Meditation

Meditation effectively offers respite from the stresses of day-to-day life, leaving you feeling calm, centred and relaxed. During a detox, it can help to reduce any side-effects you may experience (see pages 44–6) as well as encouraging a profound sense of peace, which can help balance your energy and promote good health on many levels. Some experts use a meditation to detox 'emotionally', which means letting go of negative thoughts, behaviours and emotions to replace them with those that are healthy and positive. You can meditate on your own, at home, or you can do it in a group setting, such as a yoga class, or at a local meditation centre.

The simplest way to undertake meditation at home is to focus on your breathing.

- Assume a comfortable sitting posture.
- Close your eyes, keep your spine straight, and let your shoulders drop a bit.
- Bring your attention to your abdomen, noticing it rising gently with each in breath and falling with each out breath. The rise and fall of your abdomen as you breathe will be the focus of this meditation.
- Keep the focus on your breathing – the rise and fall of the abdomen – 'being with' each in breath for its full duration and with each out breath for its full duration, rather like riding the waves of your own breathing.
- Every time you notice your attention has wandered, mentally note where it has gone, and then gently bring it back to the rise and fall of the belly as you breathe.
- Practise this for ten to 15 minutes, once or twice a day. Not only will you see where your mind 'wanders' when left to its own devices, allowing you to become more self-aware, but you will also experience profound relaxation.

There are countless other therapies that can be used in the process of detoxification, and some are better than others. Before undertaking any of them, make sure you are aware of the benefits, and the potential side-effects. Always choose a registered practitioner at a reputable clinic.

You now have all the facts you will need to start a detox. In the next section, you will find a list of 'detox superfoods' with helpful facts about their properties, to inform and inspire you. Then on pages 123–57, you'll find some detox recipes, to show you that it's not all boring brown rice and boiled cabbage. Substitute your favourite detox foods in the recipes, choose the detox aids that appeal to you the most and your detox need not be a hardship; in fact, it could be the start of an enjoyable new healthy lifestyle.

Detox superfoods A-Z

One of the best ways to encourage both the detoxifying process, and overall health, is to eat a diet rich in detox superfoods. Not only do these comprise the foundation of a healthy diet, but each of these superfoods is also rich in vitamins, minerals and other elements that work to support detoxification, and the organs involved in that process. You may be surprised to find how many different foods you can include in your detox diet, and how varied and delicious a detox diet can be.

Acai berries
Rich in omega oils
This small purple–black berry is one of the latest berry superfoods to be uncovered. It is naturally rich in omega-6 and -9 fatty acids, amino acids (the building blocks of protein), electrolytes (minerals in your blood and other body fluids that are necessary for water balance, blood acidity or pH, muscle action, and other important processes), antioxidants, fibre and vitamins A, B and E. There has been plenty of research into the health benefits of this berry, which include cleansing and detoxifying the body of infectious agents, discouraging age-related degenerative disease, improving digestive function, reducing inflammation and boosting immunity.

Almonds
Kick-start the gall bladder
Almonds are a good source of manganese, vitamin E, magnesium, calcium, copper, B vitamins and phosphorus, as well as containing good levels of the amino acid tryptophan (see under 'Figs', page 98). Studies

have found that almonds lower unhealthy cholesterol, and reduce your risk of heart disease as well as reducing blood sugar and discouraging weight gain. Almonds also help to prevent gallstones, and boost the activity of the gall bladder which works in conjunction with the liver. Traditionally, almonds were used to remove blockages and stagnation of the liver and the spleen, and to encourage healthy digestion.

Aloe vera
Powerful colon cleanser
Taken internally, the juice of the aloe vera plant is a rich source of vitamins, minerals and amino acids, as well as being a powerful detoxificant. The juice works as a laxative to cleanse the colon, and research indicates that it has been used successfully to combat fluid retention, destroy parasites, harmful bacteria and fungi in the intestinal tract, and aid digestion. It also has a strong effect on the immune system, stimulating the production of antibodies and 'killer' T-cells in the body. All cells in the body respond to aloe vera, which contains chemicals that inject themselves into the cell membranes, making them more fluid and permeable, and allowing toxins to flow out of the cells and nutrients to flow in.

Apples
Stimulate healthy digestion
Apples have been used as health tonics for centuries, and are a wonderful source of vitamins, minerals and soluble fibre. They are, for example, our richest fruit source of vitamin E, and contain good quantities of the B vitamins biotin and folic acid, which are essential for energy and digestion. Apples also contain the antioxidant vitamins A and C, and more than 12 minerals. The soluble fibre in apples is called pectin, and it helps to stimulate healthy digestion and cleanse the colon, as well as helping to remove dangerous heavy metals such as lead and cadmium. Apples are also rich in flavonoids, powerful antioxidants which can help to mop up free radicals (see page 9).

Apricots

High in antioxidants

Apricots are a wonderful source of antioxidant vitamin A, which prevents free-radical damage to cells and tissues, and is involved in the detoxification of toxins. Antioxidants are necessary for providing energy to key organs, and when they are low in the body, the liver, skin and kidneys, are unable to perform their functions. Apricots also contain other powerful antioxidants, such as lycopene, which strengthen the immune system. They have excellent levels of vitamin C (see page 58), which is essential for detoxification, as well as plenty of dietary fibre in the form of cellulose and pectin, both of which encourage cleansing and improve digestion.

Apricot kernels are rich in vitamin B17, known as 'amygdalin', which destroys cancer cells and helps to prevent their spread. They are also rich in EFAs, which enable the cell membranes to eliminate toxins from the inside to the outside of our cells, and are vital for our liver cells to cleanse the blood. Grind them and use them raw; however, don't take more than two a day.

Artichokes (globe)

Encourage healthy liver function

As well as being an excellent source of folic acid, fibre, potassium and vitamin C, artichokes contain cynarin, an acid that has been shown to encourage healthy function. They also contain a compound known as inulin, a prebiotic (see page 61) that stimulates the growth of healthy bacteria in the gut, thereby aiding digestion and encouraging healthy elimination. As a mild diuretic, artichokes encourage the body to eliminate excess water, taking toxins with it. Artichokes are a member of the thistle family – as such, they are related to milk thistle (see page 65) and share its liver-protecting qualities.

Artichokes (Jerusalem)

A rich source of prebiotics

While globe artichokes have the greatest impact on detoxification, Jerusalem artichokes also contain inulin, a prebiotic which aids the growth of beneficial bacteria in the gut. High in iron, potassium, vitamin C, phosphorus and B vitamins, Jerusalem artichokes (also known as 'sunchokes') encourage blood-sugar control and are recommended as a potato substitute for diabetics. This vegetable has been used for centuries as a digestive aid, and for liver problems and jaundice, making it an ideal addition to your detox diet.

Asparagus
Cleanses the kidneys
Asparagus contains high levels of antioxidant vitamin A, folic acid and dietary fibre, all of which are required for detoxification and healthy organ function. Asparagus is one of the richest sources of rutin (a natural substance found in plants) which together with vitamin C can help to energise and protect the body from infections by stimulating the immune system. Asparagus also has a powerful diuretic effect, which helps to encourage elimination of toxins and cleanse the kidneys. It contains prebiotics, which stimulate the growth of friendly bacteria in the gut, thus encouraging healthy digestion and elimination.

Avocados
Help to lower cholesterol
These delicious fruits are a treasure trove of nutrients, rich in folic acid, potassium, vitamin E, lutein, beta-carotene and dietary fibre. They are a great source of monounsaturated fats, which lower cholesterol and supply your body with a healthy source of fat that puts little pressure on your liver to digest. Avocados contain glutathione, an extremely powerful antioxidant that binds itself to fat-soluble toxins such as alcohol, making them water soluble and easier for the body to excrete, and also gets to them before they can begin to cause damage in the body.

Bananas
Reduce the risk of kidney stones
Bananas contain a multitude of nutrients, including vitamins C and B6, the mineral potassium and dietary fibre. Of particular interest is potassium, which suppresses calcium excretion in the urine and minimises

the risk of kidney stones, promoting healthy kidney function and elimination. Vitamin B6 is essential for antibody production and to maintain a healthy immune response, and it helps to convert carbohydrates to glucose to keep blood-sugar levels steady which is important to take pressure off your pancreas. One banana contains 16 per cent of your daily fibre requirements, which will help to keep your bowels clean, and is a good source of pectin, a soluble fibre. Bananas are an exceptionally rich source of fructo-oligosaccharide, a prebiotic that encourages the growth of healthy bacteria in the gut.

Barley

Contains both pre- and probiotics

Barley is rich in both soluble and insoluble fibre, and is an excellent prebiotic. It contains the most powerful antioxidant form of vitamin E (known as tocotrienols) and provides lignans, phytochemicals that function as antioxidants. Barley is a great source of antioxidant minerals selenium and copper, as well as manganese and phosphorus, and it is an excellent source of probiotics, which encourage healthy intestinal function. It reduces the secretion of bile acids (an excess of which can cause the formation of gallstones), increases insulin sensitivity and lowers triglycerides (blood fats). The phosphorus provided by barley plays a role in the structure of every cell in the body, encouraging them to perform at optimum level.

Barley grass

A powerful diuretic

Barley grass can be sprouted at home or purchased in health-food shops, sometimes as a powder. It is full of vitamins, minerals, enzymes and trace elements, and is particularly rich in potassium, beta-carotene and the B-complex family of vitamins. Potassium is important as it affects water balance, ensuring that toxins are efficiently excreted by the kidneys. Barley juice, from barley grass, is seven times richer in vitamin C than oranges, contains ten times more calcium than milk, and is five times richer in iron than spinach. Live enzymes contained in barley grass aid in digestion and metabolism and act as a cellular antioxidant, protecting against chemicals and radiation. Barley grass also helps to maintain a healthy pH balance in our bodies, which can become unbalanced through a poor or toxic diet.

Bean sprouts
Rich in live enzymes
Like all sprouting vegetables, bean sprouts are a great source of live enzymes, which encourage healthy digestion and elimination. Bean sprouts are rich in protein as well as antioxidant vitamins A, C and E, the B-complex vitamins, including folic acid, as well as various minerals, including calcium, iron and potassium. Most people think of mung bean sprouts when sprouts are mentioned; however, a wide variety of nuts, grains, seeds and beans can be sprouted.

Beans
A great source of soluble and insoluble fibre
All types of beans, including green, mung, pinto, kidney, cannelini, broad and soya, both fresh and dry, are excellent detoxifiers, mainly because they are very high in both soluble and insoluble fibre. Beans are high in potassium and contain good quantities of magnesium along with other vital nutrients; potassium is particularly important as it ensures that your kidneys function properly to excrete the toxins in urine. Many beans, but black beans in particular, are an excellent source of the trace mineral molybdenum, an integral component of the enzyme sulphite oxidase, which is responsible for detoxifying sulphites, a commonly used food preservative. Most beans are also rich in antioxidants – in fact, the darker the bean's coating, the higher its level of antioxidant activity. They are particularly high in antioxidant compounds called anthocyanins that protect many body systems. Beans are a great source of healthy protein, with no saturated fat.

Beetroot
Protects liver cells
Brilliantly coloured beetroot is a powerful anti-carcinogen (the result of the pigment betayanin that give beets their crimson colour), and can

help to increase the amount of oxygen our bodies can absorb by up to 400 per cent. It also contains a natural chemical that reduces inflammation, allowing every cell and organ in the body to perform more efficiently. Beetroot is rich in the antioxidant enzyme glutathione, which acts as the bodyguard for liver cells, protecting them from free-radical attack. Beetroot also improves the functions of the liver by stimulating the regeneration of liver tissue and by boosting the metabolism of dietary fats within the liver. Studies have also found that beetroot encourages immunity, helping the body to detect and eliminate abnormal cells. Beetroot is a great source of folic acid, manganese, potassium, fibre, vitamin C, iron, copper, phosphorous and magnesium, making it a truly invaluable detox superfood. It also has some chelation (see page 78) properties because it binds with heavy metals.

Blackberries
Antiviral and antibacterial properties

These dark berries are one of the richest sources of beta-carotene, the precursor to vitamin A, which is a powerful antioxidant. They also contain high levels of vitamin C and fibre, which have been shown to help reduce cancer and encourage the detoxification process. An excellent source of anthocyanins (see under 'Blueberries,' page 89), which give the berries their deep dark colour and are antioxidants, too, with a strong role to play in detoxifying the body (see page 16). Blackberries contain ellagic acid, a phenolic compound shown to have anti-carcinogenic, antiviral and antibacterial properties. They are also a good low-fat source of vitamin E and folic acid.

Blackcurrants
Excellent source of vitamin C

Thanks to the high levels of anthocyanins (see under 'Blueberries,' page 89) and vitamin C, two key antioxidants, blackcurrants have a wealth of health benefits, promoting overall good health and preventing disease. Blackcurrants have more than three times the vitamin C content of oranges and anthocyanin levels second only to some types of blueberry. Herbalists have used these berries since the Middle Ages to treat bladder stones, liver disorders and coughs, making them an ideal addition to your detox diet; today, they are widely used to prevent and treat urinary tract infections. The seeds also contain both omega-3 and -6 fatty acids, making them excellent natural anti-inflammatories.

Blueberries
Encourage healthy digestion and urinary function
Blueberries are an excellent source of vitamin C, with a small bowl containing almost 30 per cent of your daily requirements. They are rich in manganese (required for healthy liver function), dietary fibre and vitamin E. Antioxidant phytonutrients known as anthocyanins work to neutralise damage to the cells that can lead to ill health, and improve the health of your veins and arteries, ensuring that your body receives a good supply of nutrients and oxygenated blood. Blueberries contain another antioxidant compound called ellagic acid, which has been shown to help prevent cancer, as well as tannins, which act as astringents in the digestive system to reduce inflammation. In addition, they are high in the soluble fibre pectin which encourages intestinal health, and they promote urinary tract health as well, containing the same compounds found in cranberries (see page 96) that help to eliminate and prevent urinary tract infections.

Brazil nuts
Encourage the health of the thyroid gland
Brazil nuts are full of the antioxidant selenium, which works to boost immunity, as well as vitamin E. They help to protect cell membranes from free radicals and work to balance thyroid hormone metabolism. Selenium is also important for flushing heavy metals through the body by binding with them through a process called chelation, and it also supports the action of the liver. Brazil nuts are rich in calcium, as well as magnesium, manganese, copper, phosphorus and potassium. Zinc and iron are also found in good proportions in this high-mineral nut. A good source of high-quality protein.

Broccoli
Help the liver expel toxins
Like all members of the brassica family, broccoli increases levels of glutathione, a key antioxidant that helps the liver get rid of toxins. It also contains a hugely powerful antioxidant phytochemical known as sulphoraphane, which stimulates the body to produce specific detoxification enzymes which attack and destroy carcinogenic substances. In fact, the phytonutrients in broccoli direct and balance the various detoxification enzymes in the body, each of which has a protective and valuable role in encouraging our cells to clear toxins and free radicals. Broccoli is an amazing source of nutrients, including very high levels of vitamins C, K and A, as well as folic acid, dietary fibre, manganese, potassium, B vitamins, phosphorous, magnesium, protein, EFAs, iron, calcium, zinc and even a little vitamin E. It also promotes a healthy immune system, working to encourage a multitude of immune defence actions.

Brussels sprouts
All-round detoxifying aid
Like cabbage and broccoli, Brussels sprouts are a member of the brassica family, which have excellent detoxifying benefits. Chemicals contained within Brussels sprouts activate phase I of the liver detoxification process (see page 11). Just one mugful contains almost three times the recommended intake of vitamin K and almost twice the vitamin C you need. Sprouts are rich in folic acid, vitamin A, manganese, fibre, potassium, B vitamins, EFAs and iron, and there is some protein, phosphorous, magnesium, vitamin E, calcium and copper in there as well. Research has found that Brussels sprouts can inhibit the uptake of a toxin called aflatoxin, which has been linked to liver cancer, and also neutralises nitrosamines, which are produced by cigarette smoke.

Cabbage
A great detoxifier
Like Brussels sprouts and broccoli, cabbage is a powerful detoxifier, and a rich source of vitamins and minerals, including vitamin K, vitamin C,

manganese, B vitamins, EFAs, calcium – and there is also a little potassium, vitamin A and magnesium. Cabbage is high in dietary fibre, and contains a little protein as well, the amino acids of which are necessary for the liver to detox. The phytonutrients contained in cabbage optimise our bodies' ability to clear the cells of toxins. Other chemicals encourage phase II detoxification of the liver (see page 11), which detoxifies carcinogens. They also work to eliminate old and cancerous cells, as well as increasing the production of antioxidants and detoxification enzymes.

Cantaloupe

Rich in beta-carotene

This brightly coloured melon is extremely high in antioxidants vitamin C and beta-carotene (providing more than 100 per cent of the daily recommended intake for both in just one small bowlful), as well as potassium, B vitamins, folic acid and dietary fibre. Cantaloupe is a good natural diuretic, encouraging the action of the kidneys and cleansing them. The fruit is also a great source of polyphenol antioxidants, chemicals which are known to provide health benefits to the cardiovascular and immune systems.

Carrots

Restore gut imbalances and support immunity

The bright orange colour of carrots is caused by the presence of beta-carotene, a powerful antioxidant and a precursor to vitamin A. In fact, just one mugful of carrots supplies more than 600 times the suggested daily intake for this important vitamin. They are rich in vitamin K and vitamin C, and also contain dietary fibre, potassium, B vitamins, folic acid, manganese, molybdenum, phosphorus and magnesium. Chemicals contained within them are also antibacterial and antifungal, which can help to restore imbalances in the gut and support the immune system. Several studies have also found that a diet high in carrots can help to prevent lung cancer. There is some evidence, too, that carrots help to cleanse the skin from the inside out.

Cashews

Rich in essential fatty acids

Cashews contain lots of healthy proteins and monounsaturated fats, which protect the heart and make a good addition to a detox diet. They also have plenty of essential fatty acids, including phytosterols, tocopherols and sqaulene. They are rich in copper, magnesium, calcium and phosphorus, and in the amino acid tryptophan (see under 'Figs', page 98). They contain chemicals that help to prevent gallstones and gallbladder disease, and are a good source of dietary fibre, to keep your gut and digestive system working effectively and clear of toxins. As always, choose raw, unsalted nuts.

Cauliflower

Supports liver function

You may be surprised to hear that cauliflower is a detox superfood, but as a member of the brassica family, which also includes broccoli and cabbage, it contains compounds that stop enzymes from activating cancer-causing agents in the body, and increase the activity of enzymes that disable and eliminate carcinogens. What's more, cauliflower contains both glucosinolates and thiocyanates, which increase the liver's ability to neutralise potentially toxic substances. Cauliflower is rich in vitamin C, vitamin K, folic acid, B vitamins, manganese, potassium, phosphorus and magnesium, as well as containing the amino acid tryptophan, omega-3 fatty acids, some protein and lots of dietary fibre.

Celery

Maintains fluid balance and cleanses the blood

Celery is an excellent source of vitamin C, which is crucial for the detox process and supports the immune system. It is also a strong antioxidant which can prevent free-radical damage. Celery is rich in both potassium and sodium, which are necessary for fluid balance and stimulate the production of urine leading to healthy excretion of toxins and excess fluid. Its alkaline properties make it an important detoxifier, and chemicals contained within it encourage healthy digestion and assimilation of nutrients. These also work to cleanse the blood and encourage the bladder and kidneys to work effectively. It's an excellent source of fibre, and contains plenty of vitamin K, folic acid, manganese and molybdenum, as well as some B vitamins, calcium, vitamin A, phosphorus and even a little iron.

Cherries
Natural anti-inflammatories
A recent study found that cherries contain significant levels of melatonin, a hormone produced in the brain that has been associated with slowing the ageing process and the treatment of insomnia, as well as being studied as a treatment for cancer and other disorders. The red in the skin and flesh of the cherry is rich in antioxidant phytochemicals known as anthocyanins, which are important for detoxification (see under 'Blueberries,' page 89). These same antioxidants are responsible for reducing pain and inflammation. All types of cherries are rich in vitamin C, and provide potassium, folic acid, fibre, iron and magnesium; however, tart cherries appear to have more health benefits than the sweeter varieties.

Chickpeas
Aid energy production
Like all members of the bean family, chickpeas are rich in fibre and provide a source of high-quality protein. They are also a very good source of the trace mineral molybdenum, which is a key part of the enzyme sulphite oxidase, responsible for detoxifying sulphites in food. Chickpeas also have plenty of the trace mineral manganese, which is important for energy production and antioxidant defences, and they contain iron, copper, zinc and magnesium, as well as antioxidant phytochemicals known as saponins.

Chicory
Stimulates the production of bile
Also known as endive, chicory is a herb that is widely used for flavouring and as a salad vegetable. It contains good levels of dietary fibre, calcium, phosphorus, iron, beta-carotene, B vitamins, vitamin C

and even a little protein. Compounds in chicory stimulate bile production and help to cleanse the liver. It acts as a mild laxative and diuretic, which supports liver function. There is also some evidence that chicory can lower cholesterol levels in cases of fatty liver. Chicory tea and coffee make good substitutes for the real thing.

Chilli peppers

Encourage detoxification through the skin

The 'fire' of chilli peppers, and the substance that gives them their health benefits, is a chemical known as capsaicin, which is concentrated in the white membranes and seeds of red and green chilli peppers. They encourage sweating, which is a healthy way to detoxify the body, and also encourage the health of your heart as well as acting as strong anti-inflammatories and antioxidants. They are high in vitamin A, dietary fibre, potassium, iron, magnesium and vitamin C, and they help to break down mucus, which can clog the gut and respiratory system. High levels of beta-carotene promote healthy immunity, and studies have found that they work to balance blood sugar.

Cinnamon

Helps prevent urinary tract infections

This fragrant spice has been used for medicinal purposes for centuries. It contains high levels of the detox mineral manganese (see under 'Rice', page 114), as well as some dietary fibre, iron and calcium. The volatile oils that it contains have been shown to encourage the health of the heart, regulate blood-sugar levels and act as natural antibiotic and antifungal agents, particularly in the gut where overgrowths can take place. Eating it regularly can also reduce the risk of urinary tract infections. It acts as a blood-thinning agent, thereby increasing circulation and ensuring that oxygenated blood reaches every tissue in the body.

Coconuts

Contain antiviral and antibacterial fats

Coconuts contain very good levels of fibre, and are a good source of protein, vitamins and minerals, including vitamin C, B vitamins, calcium, iron, magnesium, potassium and zinc. The oil is of particular interest. Although it is a saturated fat (solid at room temperature), the fatty acids it contains are not thought to raise cholesterol levels or contribute to heart disease. About half of the fatty acids are lauric acid, which forms monolaurin in our bodies, a fat that has antiviral and antibacterial properties. Coconut oil has also been proven to be beneficial for the health of the thyroid gland, and is a traditional treatment for hypothyroidism (an underactive thyroid). By fuelling the metabolism, your body's ability to neutralise and eliminate impurities is encouraged. What's more, the lauric acid naturally kills off toxins, both those that are destructive and those that are created as by-products.

Corn

Provides a powerful antioxidant

Sweetcorn is a great detox superfood, supplying plenty of B vitamins, folic acid, dietary fibre, vitamin C, phosphorus and manganese, as well as a little protein. The carotenoid found in corn (and other bright yellow or orange fruit and vegetables) is known as beta-crytoxanthin, and it is a powerful antioxidant. Sweetcorn's fibre content is particularly important, and as a whole food it works to clear and cleanse the gut of toxins and debris, improving digestion, elimination and assimilation. And this is one vegetable that you can cook with confidence – cooking corn releases the key antioxidants, and also releases its soluble fibre. If you go for tinned, choose those brands without salt or sugar.

Courgettes

A great source of fibre

Also known as zucchini or summer squash, these fleshy vegetables are a wonderful source of manganese, vitamin C, magnesium, beta-carotene, potassium, copper, folic acid, omega-3 fatty acids, vitamin K, phosphorus, B vitamins, calcium, zinc, iron and the amino acid tryptophan, not to mention offering a good whack of fibre and a little protein. This is one superfood that should appear on any detox diet, as it's rich in phytonutrients and has anti-inflammatory benefits as well. As a good source of fibre, courgettes help to keep toxins away from the lining of the colon, which can help to prevent cancer and other diseases, and also encourage healthy elimination.

Cranberries

Discourage bacterial overgrowth in the urinary tract and kidneys

Cranberries are a popular and useful detox superfood, rich in antioxidants, and able to destroy harmful bacteria in the kidneys, bladder and urinary tract. Bacterial overgrowth can produce toxic overload, and inhibit your body's ability to detoxify properly. They are a good source of vitamin C and dietary fibre, as well as containing some manganese and vitamin K. Cranberries also seem to have some probiotic activity in the gut, inhibiting the growth of unhealthy bacteria, and a beneficial action on cholesterol levels. In comparison with 19 other common fruits, cranberries were found to have the highest level of antioxidant phenols, which mop up free radicals, in particular those affecting the liver. They may also help to cleanse the lymphatic system, which is responsible for neutralising waste products and flushing toxins from cells and body tissues.

Cucumber

An excellent natural diuretic

Cucumber is a good source of vitamin C, which aids detoxification, and their skin is rich in fibre. The high water content makes it an excellent source of hydration, while vitamin C and caffeic acid help to prevent water retention. It is an excellent natural diuretic, cleansing the kidneys, and also works as an alkalizing agent. It contains vitamin A, a little niacin (a B-complex vitamin), some calcium and iron, and lots of potassium and phosphorus. Across the centuries, cucumber has been used in the treatment of liver and pancreatic diseases.

Dandelion

Encourages the production of bile

Used both as a herb (see page 64) and a food, dandelion is a wonderfully cleansing plant, the leaves of which are rich in vitamin A (in the form of its precursor beta-carotene), B-complex vitamins, vitamin C, calcium, phosphorus, iron, sodium and lots of potassium. In fact, the dandelion ranks in the top four green vegetables for nutritional value. It is an effective diuretic, and because of its high potassium content it replaces the electrolytes that fluid removes. The leaves stimulate the production of bile, encouraging healthy digestion and helping both the liver and the gall bladder to break down fats. It also helps the liver detoxify. High in pectin, dandelion detoxifies the gastrointestinal system and encourages the health of the gut.

Elderberries
Rich in antioxidants and antiviral compounds
These small, dark berries have been used since ancient times to treat colds, flu, arthritis and constipation, among other problems. They are particularly high in antioxidants, antiviral compounds and anthocyanins (see under 'Blueberries', page 89), which encourage healthy immune function, protect against degenerative diseases and some cancers, and help to lower cholesterol; in fact, anthocyanins found in elderberries have more antioxidant capacity than either vitamin E or vitamin C. Elderberries cleanse the digestive system and promote healthy elimination from the gut and the kidneys, acting as a mild diuretic. Elderberries should never be eaten raw as they are mildly poisonous; however, cooking destroys the toxins that can cause illness.

Fennel
Strongly diuretic
This crunchy vegetable is a powerful diuretic, and helps the body to eliminate fats and to reduce intestinal bloating. It's got good levels of vitamin C, dietary fibre, potassium and manganese, and also contains folic acid, molybdenum, phosphorus, calcium, magnesium, iron and copper. The flavonoids rutin and quercitin, among others, give it a powerful antioxidant effect. The phytonutrient anethole has been shown in animal studies to reduce inflammation and prevent some cancers. Other phytochemicals in fennel support the function of the kidneys, liver and spleen.

Figs

Stimulate liver function

Figs are a good source of potassium, manganese and dietary fibre (in particular, the soluble fibre pectin), and are a fruit source of calcium. The fibre content of figs is higher than that in any other fruit or vegetable – with five figs containing more than 20 per cent of the daily recommendations for fibre – making them a good addition to any detox diet. Figs also contain tryptophan, an amino acid that promotes good sleep, encourage the brain to use glucose properly and to stimulate circulation. They have traditionally been used to enhance liver function and, as a highly alkaline food, they help to regulate the body's pH balance. They are rich in flavonoids and polyphenols, which are powerful antioxidants. Dried figs contain higher levels of naturally occurring sugars, but the other nutrients are well preserved.

Fish

The very best source of essential fatty acids

Few foods contain the exceptional nutritional value of fish, and oily fish, such as salmon, mackerel, fresh tuna and sardines, is a wonderful source of EFAs (essential fatty acids). Fish contains tryptophan (see above, under 'Figs'), vitamin D, omega fatty acids, selenium, high-quality protein, B vitamins, phosphorus and magnesium, and the protein contains an abundance of amino acids, as well as being very easily digestible. Increasing your fish intake is ideal at any time, but is particularly useful during a detox; be careful, however, to avoid fish with a high mercury content, such as swordfish, shark and king mackerel. These fish may also contain high levels of PCBs and dioxins, which are environmental pollutants.

Flaxseeds

Fantastic source of omega-3 fatty acids

Just two tablespoons of flaxseeds (also known as linseeds) contain a whopping 150 per cent of your daily recommended intake of omega-3 fatty acids. These fatty acids produce important anti-inflammatory agents, which can have a significant effect on your overall health, including protection against heart disease, cancer, diabetes and high blood pressure. They are also a great source of manganese, dietary fibre, magnesium, folic acid, copper, phosphorus and B vitamins. The high fibre content is excellent for cleansing the colon, and phytoestrogens known as 'lignans' can help to balance hormones and encourage the health of the liver and pancreas. Use the oil in dressings to get many of the superfood benefits.

Garlic

Cleanses the blood

This powerful antioxidant is an excellent blood cleanser, eliminating toxic micro-organisms and containing compounds that reduce inflammation. Allicin, one of the sulphur compounds found in garlic, is a vigorous antibacterial and antiviral agent. Garlic also increases phagocytosis, the ability of white blood cells to fight off bacterial infection (toxins).Other phytochemicals have been shown to protect against many cancers. It is very high in vitamin C, B vitamins, tryptophan and selenium, and contains very good levels of phosphorus, calcium and copper. It also strengthens the cells of your immune system. Garlic increases bile production, while enhancing digestion and reducing stomach gases. The medicinal properties and benefits of garlic are strongest when it is raw and crushed or very finely chopped.

Ginger

Stimulates digestive enzymes

This warming herb is a perfect addition to detox diets, with good levels of potassium, magnesium, copper and manganese. Across the centuries it has been used to relax and soothe the intestinal tract, and it has antioxidant and anti-inflammatory effects. It helps to stimulate digestive enzymes, which encourages healthy and efficient digestion, and is a traditional and proven modern-day remedy for travel sickness and nausea. Anti-inflammatory phytochemicals known as gingerols affect all areas of the body, and encourage the healthy function of organs. Studies have found that ginger can protect against cancer and form a part of an aggressive treatment of the disease. The warming qualities promote healthy sweating, which assists detoxification and boosts immunity.

Goji berries
A complete source of protein, and an immune system booster
Goji berries contain all 18 amino acids, making them a complete protein, as well as 21 trace minerals, linolenic acid, more beta-carotene than carrots, vitamins B1, B2, B6 and E, as well as selenium and a multitude of antioxidants. They also contain lots of iron as well as fibre, and four polysaccharides which encourage healthy immunity. These berries are rich in the phytonutrient betaine, which is used by the liver to produce choline, a compound that calms nervousness, enhances memory, promotes muscle growth and protects against fatty liver disease, as well as solavetivone, a powerful antifungal and antibacterial compound.

Grapefruit
Promotes detoxification
This tart citrus fruit is a wonderful source of vitamin C, vitamin A, potassium, folic acid and dietary fibre. Pink and red grapefruits contain lycopene, a carotenoid which has strong antioxidant qualities, and which also appears to have anti-cancer properties. What's more, limonoids, phytonutrients in grapefruit, help prevent the formation of tumours by promoting the development of an enzyme responsible for detoxification. Grapefruit also contains pectin, a soluble fibre which encourages healthy detoxification and lowers cholesterol, which can lead to clogged arteries. One of the most important roles of grapefruit is to increase the production and action of the liver's detoxification enzymes, which neutralise toxins for removal from the body. In fact, grapefruit is involved in both phases I and II of the liver detoxification process (see page 11). Like lemons (see page 103), the fruit and the juice will kick-start your liver. Go for the more brightly coloured varieties for the greatest number of nutrients.

Grapes

Cleanse the skin, liver, intestines and kidneys

Grapes are pretty much a staple in a detoxification diet, containing very high levels of flavonoids, including quercitin and resveratrol, which reduce the risk of heart disease, and help protect the body from the effects of unhealthy lifestyle choices, such as smoking and overeating saturated fats. Grapes contain plenty of manganese, vitamin C, B vitamins and potassium, and the phytonutrients they contain help prevent cancer. They are rich in powerful antioxidants (purple grape juice, from the concord grape, coming out highest in studies), and help to prevent mucus from building up in the gut. They are also excellent cleansers for the skin, liver, intestines and kidneys. Grapes enhance metabolism, which can speed up the elimination of toxins from your body, and their iron content can ensure that you feel more energetic.

Honey

Antibacterial, antifungal and antiviral activity

Raw (unpasteurised) honey contains substances that have been proven through years of research to have antibacterial, antifungal and antiviral activity, mainly due to the resins honey contains. Phytonutrients found in honey have been shown to have cancer-preventing and anti-tumour properties. Different varieties of honey possess large amounts of friendly bacteria, which encourage the health of the gut and also improve immunity. Daily consumption of honey also raises blood levels of protective antioxidant compounds. Unlike most other sweeteners, honey contains small amounts of a wide array of vitamins, minerals and amino acids, and is a great source of carbohydrates that place little stress on the digestive system, having been 'predigested' by bees. Manuka honey, from New Zealand, has particularly high levels of nutrients, as well as natural antibiotic and antifungal compounds.

Kale

Fantastic source of vitamin K

This vegetable is a powerhouse of nutrients, with more than 13 times the daily recommended intake of vitamin K, almost twice the vitamin

A in the form of beta-carotene and almost 100 per cent of daily suggested levels of vitamin C in just one mugful. It also contains manganese, copper, calcium, B vitamins, potassium, iron, magnesium, vitamin E, folic acid and phosphorus – as well as the amino acid tryptophan, good levels of protein and lots of dietary fibre, all of which add up to super detoxing. The phytonutrients kale contains help to prevent cancer, and boost the body's detoxification enzymes; they also optimise the ability of our cells to detox and to cleanse themselves. Kale's host of antioxidants provide great support for your immune system, as well as acting as a natural anti-inflammatory. The fibre content acts as a broom to sweep out your digestive system, and also to keep cholesterol levels under control.

Kiwi fruit
Contains powerful digestive enzymes
One kiwi fruit will give you almost your entire daily recommended intake of vitamin C, and kiwi is also rich in dietary fibre, potassium, copper, magnesium and even has some vitamin E. The phytonutrients in this nutritious fruit have a high antioxidant content, the result of the high levels of vitamin C and beta-carotene, which gives kiwi fruit its colour. Its high fibre content helps to bind and remove toxins from the colon, which is important for detoxing, but also for preventing colon cancer. Kiwi has powerful digestive enzymes, which can help release the nutrients from food. What's more, the edible seeds of the kiwi are rich in omega-3 essential fatty acids.

Leeks
A natural antibiotic
The humble leek is actually a very nutritious vegetable, with plenty of manganese, vitamin C, iron, folic acid and vitamin B6. Like garlic and onions, leeks belong to the allium family of vegetables, and contain many of the same beneficial compounds that lower cholesterol, reduce the risk of cancers (including cancer of the colon and ovaries), stabilise blood-sugar levels and act as a natural antibiotic. They also contain natural sulphur compounds which nourish and support the liver.

Lemons

Support and cleanse the liver

There can be no more obvious choice for a detox diet than lemons, which stimulate the release of the enzymes that are an essential part of the liver's detoxification process, encouraging it to flush out unwanted toxins. Lemon juice acts by lowering bilirubin levels (a key indicator of a damaged liver), removing heavy metals, increasing the production of bile from the liver, stimulating lymphatic flow and restoring the pH of your saliva, which in turn helps you to absorb the nutrients from the food you eat. Lemons are high in vitamin C and flavonoids, both powerful antioxidants. When the liver removes certain contaminants from the bloodstream it converts them to free radicals, which are then neutralised and mopped up by antioxidants. One group of flavonoids found in lemons, called flavonol glycosides, have a strong antibiotic effect, attacking bacterial invaders that would not only put pressure on your system, but also produce toxic waste.

Lentils

Promote healthy liver function

Lentils are an enormously nutritious pulse, high in the minerals molybdenum, manganese, iron, phosphorus and potassium. They contain the amino acid tryptophan, as well as plenty of folic acid, and both soluble fibre – which traps bile and removes it from the body – and insoluble fibre, which clears out the gut and prevents a build-up of toxins. Lentils are rich in high-quality protein and low in fat, which encourages healthy liver function. The phytonutrients contained in lentils assist in detoxification, particularly against cancer cells. All colours of lentils are equally valuable.

Lettuce

Encourages digestion

Not all lettuce is high in nutrients, but the darker-coloured varieties (rich greens, purples and yellows) will provide a wider variety of vitamins, minerals and phytonutrients. One of your best bets is Romaine or cos lettuce, of Caesar salad fame, which contains extremely high levels of vitamin K, vitamin A (as beta-carotene), vitamin C, folic acid, manganese, chromium, potassium, molybdenum, iron, B vitamins, phosphorus, calcium and even some protein, as well as the amino acid tryptophan, omega-3 fatty acids and dietary fibre. The vitamin C and beta-carotene act as powerful antioxidants, and the fibre content combined with the high water volume makes it a natural flush for your gut. Enzymes contained in this vegetable also encourage digestion and promote liver health. The chlorophyll (which gives lettuce its green colour) helps to sweep out environmental toxins (heavy metals, pesticides) and protects the liver. Lettuce can be juiced like other vegetables, too. Choose from radicchio, rocket, endive, chicory and escarole, but give iceberg a miss if you are looking for a good source of super-detox nutrients.

Limes

Increase liver enzymes

Limes contain much the same nutrients as lemons, and are equally high in the powerful antioxidant vitamin C. They are a good source of vitamin B6, potassium, folic acid and flavonoids. Limonoids, compounds found in both lemons and limes, have been shown to help fight cancers of the mouth, skin, lung, breast, stomach and colon, and act as powerful anti-carcinogens generally. Limonen, in particular, works on the body to increase the levels of liver enzymes involved in detoxifying carcinogens. Like lemons, limes are excellent liver cleansers, and help to encourage the healthy flow of bile for digestion.

Mangoes

Rich in antioxidants and enzymes

Like all brightly coloured fruit, mango is extremely high in antioxidants, in particular beta-carotene, the precursor to vitamin A. It's rich in vitamin C and its enzymes, which include magneferin, katechol oxidase and lactase, are excellent bowel cleaners, offering an ideal antidote for toxic living. They are also rich in B vitamins, folic acid (only grapes and oranges have more), calcium, magnesium, iron, zinc and potassium, as well as the amino acid tryptophan (see under 'Figs', page

98). The phenols in mango, such as quercetin, isoquercitrin, astragalin, fisetin, gallic acid and methylgallat, as well as the huge number of enzymes, have healing and cancer-preventing properties.

Maple syrup
Encourages immune function
You may not have considered something so sweet to be appropriate for detox diets; however, maple syrup is enormously nutritious and has some key health benefits. It's extremely high in manganese, an essential cofactor in enzymes that are required for energy production and antioxidant defences, and zinc, which is a powerful antioxidant. Both minerals are important for immune function.

Millet
High in insoluble fibre
This ancient grain is rich in the minerals manganese, magnesium and phosphorus, and also in the amino acid tryptophan (see under 'Figs', page 98). Magnesium, in particular, acts with more than 300 enzymes, including those that are involved in the way our bodies use glucose and secrete insulin, therefore keeping blood-sugar levels steady and preventing the risk of type 2 diabetes. Millet is high in insoluble fibre, which can help to prevent gallstones by speeding the transit time of food in your intestines and by lowering blood fats. Like many other whole grains, millet contains powerful phytonutrients that ensure health on all levels, including acting as antioxidants and preventing several forms of cancer.

Miso
Helps detoxify heavy metals
This fermented soya-bean paste originated in Japan but has become increasingly popular in the West, largely because of its excellent health-improving benefits. It is very high in tryptophan, as well as manganese, vitamin K, zinc, copper and omega-3 fatty acids; it contains good levels of protein and dietary fibre, and is a great source of vitamin B12, which tends to be lacking in vegan and vegetarian diets. Compounds found in

miso are necessary for energy production and immunity, and it is reported to help detoxify heavy metals. Miso contains strains of healthy bacteria which encourage the health of the gut.

Mushrooms (shiitake)
Promote healthy immunity

On many detox diets, mushrooms are off the menu, as they are a fungus and can contribute to the overgrowth of candida in the body. However, shiitake mushrooms are different, as they contain good levels of iron, potassium, phosphorus, selenium, vitamin D and vitamin C, as well as protein and dietary fibre. They also contain an active compound called lentinan, which encourages the health of the immune system and has anticancer activity. Another compound in this mushroom, known as eritadenine, lowers cholesterol. Shiitake mushrooms contain potent antioxidants and a compound that works to soften the stools, preventing constipation and a build-up of toxins in the intestines.

Nettles
Flush the kidneys

Stinging nettles may not seem like an obvious addition to any menu, but they are rich in iron, phytonutrients, vitamins C, D and K, as well as calcium, magnesium, potassium and silica (required for cell rejuvenation). Eating them fresh may be a step too far, but young leaves can be juiced or cooked to produce a delicious broth (see page 127), or added to soups and stews. Nettles are a natural diuretic, flushing the kidneys and promoting the elimination of liquid waste, and are often used as a urinary tract tonic. A number of studies have found that nettles lower blood-sugar levels, and the tannins they contain act as an astringent to draw out toxins from the cells for removal.

Oats
Balance blood-sugar levels

Oats are an excellent source of fibre, and contain high levels of manganese, selenium, tryptophan, phosphorus, B vitamins, magnesium and even protein. In fact, oats have a higher concentration of calcium, protein, magnesium, iron, zinc, copper, manganese, thiamine and vitamin E than other whole-grain foods such as wheat and rye. Studies have found that they lower cholesterol levels and reduce the risk of heart disease. They also contain antioxidants, known as avenanthramides, which prevent free radicals from damaging healthy cholesterol. Oats are a very good source of selenium, which is necessary for the potent antioxidant glutathione to work its magic, in particular on the liver, lungs, colon and heart. They help to keep your blood-sugar levels steady, which is crucial during a detox programme, and also soothe the digestive system. Their high levels of soluble and insoluble fibre help to keep the intestines clear and promote healthy digestion and assimilation of nutrients.

Olives and olive oil
Activate the secretion of bile
The rustic olive and its oil are powerful antioxidants and prevent cholesterol from being transformed into a harmful free radical. Olive oil activates the secretion of bile and pancreatic hormones, and lowers the incidence of gallstone formation by flushing the gall bladder and bile duct, which have accumulated large amounts of bile. When bile is excreted, the residues are passed through the intestines. What's more, the phytonutrient oleic acid, found in olives and olive oil, assists the liver to detoxify cholesterol. Olives are rich in iron, vitamin E and copper, and are a good source of dietary fibre. They are concentrated in monounsaturated fats, which protect our cells from damage. They also contain polyphenols and flavonoids, phytonutrients that have anti-inflammatory properties. Green olives are unripe olives, and if they are traditionally treated to remove their bitterness, they are as healthy as the darker brown, purple and black ripe olives. Olive oil comes in grades, the best for your health being 'extra virgin' which comes from the first pressing of the olives.

Onions
Excellent probiotics
Onions are rich in the antioxidant quercetin, which helps to protect against free-radical damage and a number of cancers, including colon

cancer. Quercetin and other flavonoids also work to kill harmful bacteria. They are excellent probiotics, enhancing the activity of the healthy intestinal bacteria known as gut flora, and have good antiviral properties too. They are rich in chromium, vitamin C, manganese, dietary fibre, molybdenum, B vitamins, folic acid, potassium, phosphorus and copper, as well as the amino acid tryptophan (see under 'Figs', page 98). Onions are a great way to lower blood sugar by decreasing the amount of free insulin available, by occupying sites in the liver where insulin is inactivated. One important property of onions is their ability to break up mucus, which can line the membranes of your gastrointestinal tract and respiratory system (see page 23). Reducing this build-up will result in overall better health on many levels.

Oranges

Inactivate toxins and encourage their excretion

Favoured for their extremely high vitamin C content, and a good source of a dietary fibre, oranges also contain folic acid, potassium, vitamin A (in the form of beta-carotene) and even some calcium. They are rich in phytonutrient flavonoids known as flavanones, which are powerful antioxidants, have been shown to lower high blood pressure and cholesterol, and to have an strong anti-inflammatory effect. Many of the most important flavonoids are found in the pith and inside skin, so eating the whole fruit rather than just drinking the juice is important to gain optimum benefit. Like limes and lemons, oranges contain limonoids which have been shown to help fight cancers of the mouth, skin, lung, breast, stomach and colon. In particular, one limonoid known as limonene has the ability to inactivate toxins and encourage their excretion from the body. The high dietary fibre content helps to grab toxins away from the lining of the gut, preventing build-up.

Papayas

An impressive digestive aid

Just one papaya contains three times your daily recommended intake of vitamin C, and good levels of folic acid, potassium, vitamin A (as beta-carotene), vitamin E and vitamin K. They are also rich in dietary fibre which works with the above nutrients to protect your heart and reduce the risk of colon cancer. Papayas contain a digestive enzyme, papain, which is an impressive digestive aid, encouraging the digestion of proteins, and also helping to break down mucus in the digestive tract. They are also excellent probiotics, and contain phytonutrients that have probiotic activity. Research has shown that papain can be effective in fighting cancer as it breaks down a protein substance called fibrin, found in all cancer cells. Papaya also helps the body to produce glutathione, essential for detoxification of the liver (see page 61).

Parsley

Encourages the action of the kidneys

This common herb is an excellent detoxifier, acting as a diuretic to help the kidneys to flush out toxins and containing phytonutrients that support the liver. It has also been shown to inhibit the re-absorption of salt into the body tissues which increases the herb's activity as a diuretic. Parsley is rich in antioxidants, including vitamin C, which supports and cleanses the body at cell level as well as boosting immunity. The bright green colour comes from chlorophyll, which cleanses the bowels, liver and lungs. Other key nutrients include vitamin K, beta-carotene, folic acid and iron. This herb contains volatile oils and flavonoids, which have a host of health benefits, including antioxidant and anti-carcinogenic activity.

Peaches

Improve liver function

These succulent fruits are rich in potassium, and also contain plenty of vitamins C and A (in the form of beta-carotene), both of which are potent antioxidants (see page 16). Peaches have diuretic and laxative properties, and are involved in the stimulation of digestive juices. They contain some calcium, magnesium, phosphorus and folic acid, and are a very good source of dietary fibre, particularly if eaten with their skins. Peaches help the liver to carry out the digestive processes by increasing the production of bile so that it favours the digestion of fat, in much the same way as dandelion or chicory. Peaches also contain some selenium, which is one of the minerals involved in removing heavy metal toxins from the body (see page 59).

Peanuts

Help to prevent gallstones

Once frowned upon for their high fat content, peanuts are now known to be a very nutritious nut, and an important part of a healthy diet. They are rich in manganese, B vitamins and copper, as well as in protein and the amino acid tryptophan (see under 'Figs', page 98). They are a great source of monounsaturated fats, which reduces the risk of heart disease considerably. They provide an antioxidant known as resveratrol, found in grapes (see page 101), which has a specific action on the cardiovascular system. They also contain oleic acid, the healthy fat found in olive oil, and they are as rich in other antioxidants as many fruits. They also work to prevent gallstones. Peanuts must, however, be raw and unsalted, or they will put pressure on the liver.

Pears

Encourage intestinal health

The extremely high fibre content of pears makes them an excellent detoxifier, clearing the gut of debris and encouraging healthy elimination and assimilation, as well as intestinal health. Pears are considered to be a hypoallergenic fruit because they tend to cause fewer reactions than other types, making them easy on the system and digestion. They are rich in vitamin C, vitamin K and copper, making them a great source of antioxidants.

Peas

Promote balanced energy levels

Green peas are eaten so commonly it's hard to believe they could be detox superfoods, but they most certainly are! Not only are they an excellent source of good-quality protein, but they are also rich in vitamin K, manganese, vitamin C, dietary fibre, B vitamins, folic acid, beta-carotene, phosphorus, magnesium, copper, iron, zinc and potassium, as well as dietary fibre and the amino acid tryptophan. They are essential for bone and heart health, encourage balanced energy levels, promote overall health and, in particular, help the body deal with environmental pollution and toxic chemicals. They also enhance immune function and help to inhibit the formation of cancer-causing compounds in the body. Fresh or frozen peas are the most nutritious.

Peppers

Rich in antioxidants

With their vibrant colours, bell peppers are a wonderful source of the antioxidants vitamin C and beta-carotene, providing three times the recommended daily intake of vitamin C and 100 per cent of the recommended daily intake of vitamin A – in just one small bowlful. They contain lots of dietary fibre as well as molybdenum, vitamin K, manganese, folic acid, potassium, B vitamins, vitamin E, copper and the amino acid tryptophan. Red peppers contain lycopene (see under 'Tomatoes', page 119), a carotenoid which has been strongly linked with cancer prevention and treatment. Green peppers are an abundant source of the phytonutrient luteolin, a flavonoid that has antioxidant, anti-inflammatory and anti-tumour properties. Fibre found in peppers can help to reduce the amount of contact that colon cells have with cancer-causing toxins.

Pine nuts

Stimulate hormone activity

Pine nuts contain more high-quality protein than any other nut or seed, and have a high concentration of monounsaturated fat, which protects the cardiovascular system and also puts less pressure on the liver than other types of fat. They contain vitamins B and D, the anti-oxidants vitamin A and C, as well as the minerals phosphorus, copper, zinc, calcium, selenium and potassium. They also contain very high levels of iron, which is a key component of red blood cells. Pine nuts are the only natural source of pinoleic acid, which stimulates hormones and helps diminish your appetite, and they have a very high concentration of oleic acid, which aids the liver in eliminating harmful triglycerides from the body.

Pineapple

Contains protein-digesting enzymes

Pineapple is an excellent source of a variety of different nutrients, including vitamin C, B vitamins, manganese and copper, as well as offering a good dose of dietary fibre. It contains bromelain, a complex blend of chemicals, which includes protein-digesting enzymes, anti-inflammatory agents, anti-coagulants (natural blood-thinners) and overall help for the digestive system, including the colon and liver. The high levels of vitamin C provide antioxidant production, and manganese and B vitamins (in particular thiamine) help to improve energy levels. Eat fresh, raw pineapple whenever possible, as the tinned and cooked fruit loses much of its nutritional value.

Pistachios

Excellent source of fibre

These delicious kernels have the lowest fat content of any nut, and much of the fat they do contain is healthy monounsaturated fat. They are a great source of protein and offer significant amounts of four vital minerals: magnesium, calcium, iron and potassium. They also have the highest fibre content among nuts, which makes them an ideal detox superfood. Both the purple skins and the green nuts themselves contain anthocyanins, which are key antioxidants and anti-inflammatories. Pistachios also contain more lutein (see under 'Raspberries', page 114) than a glass of orange juice. They are rich in B vitamins and contain good levels of copper, as well as the amino acid arginine, which helps to dilate blood vessels and increase the blood flow.

Plums

Natural laxatives

High in antioxidants vitamin C and beta-carotene, plums also contain B vitamins (in particular riboflavin) as well as potassium and dietary fibre. Phytonutrients known as phenols act as antioxidants, and are particularly good at neutralising a type of free radical which can lead to a build-up of triglycerides and cholesterol. Only wild blueberries and cranberries contain more phenols than plums. Plums are also a natural source of sorbitol, a sugar alcohol that acts as a natural laxative. They come in a variety of different colours, but all are healthy and contain different combinations of nutrients.

Pomegranates
Excellent source of antioxidants
The seeds, fruit and juice of this fruit are rich in antioxidants, and research has found that pomegranates can lower cholesterol levels, improve the flow of oxygen to the heart and prevent several cancers, such as breast and prostate. It is highly anti-inflammatory, and encourages the healthy action of the gut. One pomegranate has about 40 per cent of the recommended daily vitamin C requirement for adults, along with folic acid, fibre, potassium, niacin, and vitamins A and E.

Pumpkin seeds
Supporting the kidneys
Very nutritious, with good levels of manganese, magnesium, phosphorus, iron, copper, zinc, vitamin K, the amino acid tryptophan and plenty of protein, pumpkin seeds also contain omega oils and carotenoids that have been proven to promote prostate health. They also contain phytosterols that lower cholesterol, as well as offering a good source of monounsaturated fats. Pumpkin seeds can support the kidneys and prevent kidney stones and are a natural laxative, keeping toxins moving out of the body.

Quinoa
Excellent source of omega oils
This easily digested, cleansing grain is, in fact, a seed and a fantastic source of protein (it's one of the few plant foods that contains all of the essential amino acids, making it a complete protein). It also contains a wide range of omega oils, vitamins and minerals, including manganese, magnesium, iron, copper and phosphorus. Quinoa protects against heart disease and encourages blood vessels to relax, improving circulation. The liver requires protein to detox, so quinoa makes a good addition to any detox diet. Quinoa contains both soluble and insoluble

fibre, which cleanses the gut, and encourages healthy assimilation of nutrients.

....

Raspberries
Antibacterial and antifungal action
Like all berries, raspberries are a great source of antioxidants, and are also rich in manganese, vitamin C, dietary fibre, folic acid and other B vitamins, potassium, magnesium, omega-3 fatty acids and copper. One antioxidant contained in raspberries is ellagic acid, which prevents damage to cell membranes and other body structures caused by free radicals. Raspberries also contain flavonoids known as anthocyanins which have antibacterial and antifungal actions. Like blueberries, raspberries contain lutein, which is essential for healthy eyesight, and the soluble fibre pectin which encourages healthy digestion and absorption of nutrients.

....

Rice (brown)
Encourages healthy elimination of toxins
Brown rice is a staple in any detox diet, as its high fibre content means it cleanses the intestines as it passes through. It also helps to stabilise blood-sugar levels. Brown rice is an excellent source of manganese, selenium, magnesium, iron, B vitamins and the amino acid tryptophan. It contains some protein, and is a very good source of complex carbohydrate. Manganese in particular is a key component of a very important antioxidant enzyme called superoxide dismutase (SOD), which protects the body from free radicals and toxins. The selenium content of brown rice is important for the production of glutathione (see page 61), which the liver requires to detoxify a large number of harmful toxins. There are numerous cardiovascular benefits to brown rice, which protects against heart disease and helps to ensure healthy circulation, and which also encourages healthy elimination of toxins from the body. Its phytonutrient content is equal to or even higher than in some fruits and vegetables. Finally, its plant lignans (a type of phytonutrient) are converted in the gut into substances that are believed to help protect against breast and other hormone-related cancers.

Rye
Wonderful internal cleanser
This flavourful grain is rich in manganese, selenium, phosphorus and magnesium, and is an excellent source of dietary fibre. Rye fibre contains non-cellulose polysaccharides, which have a great capacity to bind with water, making rye one of the best internal cleansers around. As a whole grain, rye also prevents gallstones, lowers the risk of diabetes and protects against cardiovascular disease and some types of cancers.

Seaweed
Strengthens the digestive tract
Seaweed is an extremely nutritious food, offering the greatest number of minerals in any single food. It helps to alkalinise the blood and strengthens the digestive tract. Seaweed contains a huge amount of iodine, which promotes healthy thyroid function, as well as vitamin K, folic acid, magnesium, calcium, iron and the amino acid tryptophan. It is a good source of lignans, which are plant compounds associated with protecting against cancer. Studies have found that seaweed contains chemicals that process toxins to a less harmful form, including heavy metals, radiation and pollution. It also acts as a natural antibiotic, which can remove unhealthy pathogens from your bloodstream and gut. The brilliantly coloured seaweeds are also an excellent source of flavonoids, carotenoids and other phytonutrients.

Sesame seeds
Natural anti-inflammatories
One of the most prolific nutrients in sesame seeds is copper, a powerful antioxidant (see page 16) and a known anti-inflammatory. Sesame seeds also contain very good levels of calcium, manganese, phosphorus, iron, B vitamins, zinc, magnesium and dietary fibre. Phytosterols in these seeds lower cholesterol, and the high zinc levels encourage healthy bones. Both methionine and tryptophan, the amino acids which encourage healthy liver and kidney function, are found in large amounts in sesame seeds; in fact, sesame seeds have been shown to protect the liver cells from alcohol and other chemicals. They are also a

rich source of both soluble and insoluble fibre, keeping the gut clean, clear and healthy.

....

Soya

Balances hormonal activity in women

Soya beans are the most widely grown pulse in the world, and form the basis of the diet in many cultures. These beans, which can be used to make soya milk, yoghurt and tofu, are rich is many nutrients, including molybdenum, manganese, high-quality protein, iron, omega-3 fatty acids, phosphorus, vitamin K, magnesium, copper, B vitamins and potassium, as well as the amino acid tryptophan. They are a very good source of dietary fibre – both soluble and insoluble – and also contain some calcium, making soya products a suitable alternative to cow's milk and dairy produce in a non-dairy diet. Soya lowers blood pressure and cholesterol, and acts as an antioxidant. It's also an excellent source of phytoestrogens, which can help to balance hormonal activity in women, and thereby affect liver health. Dairy produce causes the body to produce mucus (see page 23), particularly in the digestive tract, which not only feeds pathogens and cancer cells, but also prevents healthy elimination and assimilation. Soya is an ideal alternative to dairy, and its wholegrain activity encourages good digestive health. Try to choose organic soya products wherever possible, as a lot of soya is genetically modified.

....

Spinach

Helps clear out environmental toxins

More than 23 different flavonoids have been discovered in spinach, which work as antioxidants and anti-cancer agents. It is an excellent source of vitamin K, which is required for bone health (in fact, just one mugful of cooked spinach offers over 1,000 per cent of the daily recommended intake of this key vitamin), as well as double the recommended intake of beta-carotene, lots of manganese, folic acid, magnesium, iron, vitamin C, B vitamins, calcium, potassium, copper, phosphorus, zinc, vitamin E, omega-3 fatty acids and selenium. Spinach is a great source of dietary fibre and the amino acid tryptophan, as well as offering a little protein. The chlorophyll contained in spinach helps to clear out environmental toxins, such as heavy metals and pesticides, and also helps to protect the liver from damage.

Squash
Wonderful source of beta-carotene
These brightly coloured vegetables are rich in beta-carotene, providing more than 150 per cent of your daily recommended intake in just one mugful. Squash also contains vitamin C, potassium, good levels of dietary fibre, manganese, folic acid and other B complex vitamins, copper, omega-3 fatty acids and the amino acid tryptophan. There are also antioxidants, including an orange–red carotenoid known as beta-cryptoxanthin which reduces the risk of lung cancer. Because squash is rich in sodium, it is an excellent alkalising treatment for acidosis of the liver, which is the result of depressed liver function.

Strawberries
Powerful antioxidants
Strawberries contain phytonutrients known as phenols, which have heart-protective, anti-cancer and anti-inflammatory benefits. They help to prevent the brain from oxidative stress, and are an excellent source of vitamins C and K, manganese, fibre and iodine, as well as containing potassium, folic acid, B vitamins, omega-3 fatty acids, magnesium and copper. The anthocyanins (see under 'Blueberries, page 89) in strawberries provide the bright red colour, serve as powerful antioxidants that improve health and protect against degenerative diseases.

Sunflower seeds
Important detoxifiers
Nutritious sunflower seeds contain almost an entire day's recommended intake of vitamin E in just one handful, as well as B vitamins, manganese, magnesium, copper, selenium, phosphorus and the amino acid tryptophan. They are rich in essential fatty acids (EFAs), which promote cardiovascular health and act as anti-inflammatories. Phytosterols in the seeds lower cholesterol, and the high selenium content

makes them excellent antioxidants and important detoxifiers, as selenium is required for glutathione, which is used by the liver to detoxify toxic chemicals (see page 61).

Sweet potatoes

Help remove heavy metals

This robust vegetable is a great source of beta-carotene, vitamin C, manganese, copper, B vitamins, potassium, iron and dietary fibre. It contains many antioxidants and anti-inflammatory agents, as well as compounds known as phytochelatins that can remove heavy metals from the body by binding to them and encouraging their excretion.

Tea (green)

Reduces the risk of gallstones

Green tea is rich in flavonoids, including catechins, which are known for their anticancer and antioxidant effects. Green tea has been found, in numerous studies, to help protect against most cancers, heart disease and stroke. While green tea does contain a little of the stimulant caffeine, it is offered in a pure, natural form which does not create or leave toxins and appears to be less damaging to health. Green tea lowers triglycerides in the body, thins the blood and helps to keep the arteries clear, which promotes healthy circulation and, through that, detoxification and elimination. It also reduces the risk of gallstones and biliary tract cancers, encouraging the health of the liver and gall bladder. A recent study also found that it protects against kidney disease. Green tea protects the liver's cells and at the same time boosts the immune system. Its antioxidants have been proven to protect the liver from the damaging effects of alcohol, cigarette smoking and other toxins. Moreover, one research project reported that green tea might help prevent the growth of cancer cells in the liver and other organs of the body.

Tofu

Rich in plant oestrogens

Tofu is an extremely nutritious, protein-rich food that is made from the curds of soya milk. It is rich in the amino acid tryptophan (see under

'Figs', page 98), which is necessary for healthy liver function and detox-ification, and it also contains manganese, iron, omega-3 fatty acids, selenium, copper, phosphorus, calcium and magnesium. It is rich in phytoestrogens, which can encourage hormonal balance and help to prevent the symptoms of PMS and menopause, as well as many female cancers. It's a good source of iron, which is required for energy, and also offers antioxidant protection. The liver requires protein for detoxifica-tion, and this makes an excellent substitute for animal proteins, which can ferment in the bowel, feeding pathogens and clogging the gut.

Tomatoes
Essential for colon health
Tomatoes, particularly cooked, are a rich source of the antioxidant carotenoid lycopene, which is believed to help prevent a variety of dis-eases, including cancer and heart disease. Lycopene is also essential for the health of your colon, which is crucial for healthy digestion and elimination and for the assimilation of nutrients. Tomatoes are rich in vitamin C, beta-carotene, vitamin K and molybdenum, and contain potassium, manganese, fibre, chromium, B vitamins, copper, magne-sium, iron, phosphorus, vitamin E and the amino acid tryptophan. The carotenoids in tomatoes also encourage the production and activity of detoxification enzymes in the liver. Tomato juice has also been found to be a natural anti-inflammatory due to its high antioxidant levels.

Turmeric
Encourages liver enzymes
This delightful spice is a perfect complement to any detox diet, and studies have found that it encourages the detoxification enzymes of the liver, which improve function and help to rid the body of toxins that could potentially lead to cancer. It contains plenty of iron and man-ganese, and is a good source of vitamin B6, dietary fibre and potassium. The volatile oil that turmeric contains is a powerful anti-inflammatory and encourages the health of the gut. The principal chemical component of turmeric is curcumin. In addition to its liver detox use, it is a natural antiviral agent and stimulates the gall bladder for bile

production. Curcumin also prevents alcohol and other toxins from being converted into compounds that may be harmful to the liver.

Walnuts
Support the immune system

Walnuts are a great source of omega-3 fatty acids, with just six to eight offering almost 100 per cent of your daily recommended intake. They also contain manganese, copper and the amino acid tryptophan, and are an excellent source of protein. Walnuts contain an antioxidant known as ellagic acid, which supports the immune system and acts as an anticancer agent. In fact, they have one of the highest antioxidant contents of all of the tree nuts. They are a good source of mono-unsaturated fats, which have a protective effect on the cardiovascular system as well as lowering cholesterol. These fats also improve circulation, which encourages healthy elimination and a good supply of oxygenated blood to the cells. One study found that walnuts protect the arteries after eating a high-fat meal, which has been attributed to their omega-3 oils. Finally, walnuts are a source of the amino acid arginine, which helps the liver detoxify ammonia, a waste product in the body.

Water
Essential for life and all detoxification processes

One of the most important elements of any detox diet and, indeed, healthy living, is water. Not only is water essential for hydration of the tissues and healthy elimination of toxins from the body, but there is not a single body function that does not depend upon it. It is actually nutritious, too. Good-quality water contains lots of essential minerals and trace elements, such as calcium and magnesium, as it percolates through the earth's surface in the form of rainfall and becomes 'mineralised'. Well water and natural mineral waters are your best bet, as water from the tap tends to lose its mineral content due to processing. What's more, tap water, even when it is filtered, can contain traces of pesticides, hormones (from birth-control pills and HRT) and other types of medication, including painkillers, which are not advisable at any stage of your life, but most particularly not on a detox diet.

Watercress
Cleanses the liver and kidneys

A versatile vegetable, watercress can be eaten raw in salads, used as a base for pesto (see page 152) or cooked as a soup to encourage healthy elimination of wastes from the body. Several studies have found that it assists in cleansing the liver and kidneys by acting as a natural diuretic, encourages the health of the bladder and urinary tract and promotes healthy digestion. With its high vitamin C content, watercress supports the immune system, and is a rich source of iron to provide energy and oxygenated blood. Along with vitamin C, other antioxidants include vitamin E, which mops up free radicals and other toxins. Some research has found that watercress increases the detox enzymes in the body, acting especially on certain toxins. In particular one study found that when smokers were given 170g of watercress a day, they excreted higher than average levels of known carcinogens in their urine.

Watermelon
An excellent purifier

Brightly coloured watermelon is a great source of vitamin C, beta-carotene, B vitamins, potassium and magnesium, and its high water content makes it a great purifier, encouraging elimination and helping to flush toxins from the body. It's rich in antioxidants, and contains a concentrated source of the carotenoid lycopene, which has been widely studied for its antioxidant and cancer-preventing activity in the body. It's also a powerful natural diuretic, and can help to reduce inflammation throughout the body. Blend it with its seeds for an even greater health kick.

Yoghurt (live)
Promotes the growth of healthy bacteria in the gut

Although dairy produce is normally a no-no on a detox diet, live yoghurt is an exception to the rule, and an important one at that. Live yogurt contains probiotics that reduce intestinal inflammation and fungal infections, and eliminate unhealthy bacteria that damage the walls of the gut. Apart from protein, which is required by the liver for detoxification, yoghurt contains good levels of calcium, potassium and magnesium, B vitamins and iodine (which encourage healthy thyroid function and metabolism). Make sure you eat plain live yoghurt, though, without any sugar or fruit added, as they can interfere with your detox and the activity of the healthy bacteria contained in the yoghurt. Goat's and sheep's yoghurt are the best option, as they are easier to digest than live cow's milk yoghurt.

Recipes

You may be a diva in the kitchen and have lots of your own ideas, but if you need a little inspiration, you might find the following recipes useful. They can inspire you to create your own combinations of important detox foods to produce the ideal detox menu. You are free to eat as much or as little as you wish on the *Perfect Detox* programme; indeed, the most important thing is that you get the necessary balance of nutrients. Start with a small portion and give yourself a little time before taking a second helping, to allow your brain to register when you are full. Most of the recipes below offer several portions to allow you to serve more than one person (if required) or to provide you with a few meals for the coming days. Everything apart from salads can be frozen for future use, too, and you may want to use leftovers as nutritious snacks between meals.

Just a word on measures – by and large you'll find really precise measures in these recipes when something strong is being used; otherwise there's a lot of flexibility as you will see. It's often more convenient to use something like a mug as a measure, but this means a standard one, holding about 250–300ml of liquid. If some of the ingredients are unfamiliar and you're not sure how to make them up – perhaps quinoa, for instance – most brands have clear instructions on their packaging.

Breakfast

Baked apples

4 green organic apples
2 handfuls of raisins or sultanas
8 chopped almonds
2 pinches of ground cinnamon
1 tablespoon of maple syrup
To serve:
live yoghurt
drop of pure vanilla essence
or oatmeal
unsweetened rice milk

This recipe will serve four, so you can use it for desserts later on in the week, or as a tasty snack – they are delicious cold. Preheat the oven to 180°C / gas mark 4. Slice about 1cm off the tops of the apples, and put the tops to one side. Remove the cores without breaking through the bottom of the apple. Blend together the raisins or sultanas, chopped almonds, cinnamon and maple syrup in a food processor. Stuff this mixture equally into the apples, and top up with water. Cover each apple with its top, and then bake for 30–40 minutes until soft. Serve with live yoghurt with a dash of pure vanilla essence mixed in, or warm oatmeal made with unsweetened rice milk.

Maple millet

5 tablespoons of millet
pinch of sea salt
To serve:
2 tablespoons of maple syrup
125ml unsweetened brown rice milk

Stir together 250ml of water with the millet and sea salt. Cook for 25 minutes on a low heat until the water is absorbed. Stir in the maple syrup and brown rice milk, and serve. This is also delicious served cold with fresh fruit purée (see page 151).

Apple flaxseed pancakes

1 egg
2 tablespoons of grated apple
4 tablespoons of flaxseeds
2 tablespoons of honey
olive oil
To serve:
pinch of cinnamon
1 tablespoon of grated apple
plain live yoghurt

Whisk together the egg, grated apple, flaxseeds, honey and 2 table-spoons of water. Heat a little olive oil in a frying pan, and pour the batter into the centre. Cook for 3 to 4 minutes, then carefully lift and turn over, repeating on the other side. To serve, sprinkle with cinnamon, grated apple and a smattering of plain live yoghurt.

Peanut butter and banana corn quesadillas

corn tortillas
unsalted, unsweetened peanut butter
sliced bananas
cinnamon
To serve:
apple purée
or plain live yoghurt

Simply spread corn tortillas with peanut butter (or any other raw nut butter), top with sliced bananas and a sprinkle of cinnamon, and place another tortilla on top. Slice into quarters, and serve with fresh apple purée or a little plain live yoghurt.

Fruity quinoa

250g quinoa
apple or grape juice
1 handful of dried chopped apricots
1 handful of sultanas
1 handful of dried or fresh cranberries
1 handful of dried blueberries, pineapple, mango or apple
2 drops of pure vanilla essence
cinnamon
To serve:
unsweetened rice milk
honey (optional)
or lightly toasted flaxseeds
almonds

Make up 250g quinoa following the instructions on the box, but replacing water with apple or grape juice. Halfway through cooking stir in the apricots, sultanas, cranberries and a good handful of any other dried fruits that strike your fancy, such as blueberries, pineapple, mango or apple. Stir in the vanilla essence and a pinch of cinnamon. Cook until all of the liquid is absorbed, and serve with unsweetened rice milk and a little honey (if desired), or sprinkle with lightly toasted flaxseeds or raw slivers of almonds.

Lunch

Nettle soup

2 tablespoons of olive oil
2 medium onions, finely sliced
1 large carrot, chopped
2 celery sticks, chopped
2 large garlic cloves, crushed
10 good handfuls of nettles
1 litre of good-quality, low-sodium vegan stock
black pepper
nutmeg
a pinch of sea salt
3 tablespoons of cooked brown rice or 3 brown rice cakes
2 tablespoons of plain live yoghurt
To serve:
plain live yoghurt
chopped fresh chives

In the bottom of a large saucepan, heat the olive oil, onions, carrot and celery. Add the crushed garlic cloves and cook the mixture, stirring frequently, until everything has softened. Rinse the nettles (use gloves to pick them!), and add to the saucepan with the stock. Bring to the boil, and simmer for 10 minutes. Season with black pepper, a grating of nutmeg and a pinch of sea salt. Then purée the soup in a liquidiser with the cooked brown rice or the rice cakes, broken up. Return it to the heat and stir in the plain live yoghurt. Serve immediately, with an extra swirl of yoghurt and a sprinkle of chopped fresh chives.

Stuffed bell peppers

4 peppers
2 teaspoons of sesame oil
2 garlic cloves, minced
2 mugfuls of cooked brown rice
1 mugful of cooked cannellini beans
2 finely chopped spring onions
1 teaspoon of ground coriander
1 tablespoon of fresh salsa (shop-bought)
a pinch of sea salt
ground black pepper

This recipe will serve two to four as it is, so you can put some aside for lunches later in the week if you wish.

Preheat the oven to 200°C/gas mark 6. Cut the tops off the peppers and remove the seeds and pith; set the peppers to one side and reserve the tops. Mix together the sesame oil, garlic, brown rice, cannellini beans, spring onions, coriander and salsa. Add a pinch of sea salt, and ground black pepper to taste. Stuff mixture into the peppers, and place them on to a baking sheet with their tops back on. Bake for 25 minutes, and serve.

Ratatouille

1 small aubergine
2 courgettes
2 small onions
1 red pepper
1 green pepper
1 yellow pepper
3 tablespoons of olive oil
2 garlic cloves, chopped
1 teaspoon of red wine vinegar
2 tablespoons of oregano

2 x 400g tins of chopped tomatoes
1 tablespoon of freshly chopped basil
2 bay leaves,
a pinch of sea salt
freshly ground black pepper

Preheat the oven to 200°C /gas mark 6. Chop the vegetables into bite-sized chunks. Heat a medium ovenproof pan with the olive oil, and then add the garlic. Simmer for a few minutes, then add the chopped vegetables, red wine vinegar, oregano, tomatoes, basil, bay leaves, sea salt and plenty of freshly ground black pepper. Cover and cook in the oven for 45 minutes, stirring occasionally. The vegetables will be soft and the ratatouille will be robustly stewlike; remove the bay leaves before serving.

Vegetable curry

1 tablespoon of olive oil
½ a medium-sized aubergine cut into sticks
2 small carrots cut into sticks
3 handfuls of frozen or fresh peas
200g of green beans
1 medium-sized sweet potato, peeled and cut into chunks
8 tablespoons of freshly grated coconut
2 hot green chilli peppers
2 tablespoons of poppy seeds
2 pinches of sea salt
3 chopped medium-sized tomatoes
2 tablespoons of live yoghurt
1 teaspoon of nitrate-free garam masala
To serve:
fresh coriander

In a medium-sized saucepan, warm the olive oil, and add the aubergine, carrots, peas, green beans and sweet potato. Cover and cook for 4 minutes on medium heat, until the vegetables are just tender. Meanwhile, liquidise the grated coconut, chilli peppers, poppy seeds and sea salt with 150ml of water until smooth. When the vegetables are cooked, add this spice paste, along with the tomatoes, live yoghurt, garam masala and 150ml more water. Bring to the boil and simmer for 3–4 minutes. Serve garnished with fresh coriander.

Marinated vegetable kebabs

For the marinade:
your choice of fresh herbs
3 tablespoons of olive oil
3 tablespoons of red or white grape juice
2 tablespoons of freshly squeezed lemon juice
sea salt
freshly ground pepper
For the kebabs:
aubergine chunks
sweet potato or squash squares
peppers
cherry tomatoes
courgettes

The secret to this is to use as many fresh herbs as you can in the marinade for the vegetables. Anything goes – choose from chervil, basil, rosemary, thyme, parsley, mint, coriander or all of the above. Chop them well. Mix the olive oil, red or white grape juice and freshly squeezed lemon juice in a large bowl, and add a good sprinkling of sea salt and freshly ground pepper. Then drop in the herbs, stir together and set to one side.

Chop your vegetables into bite-size chunks. Blanch everything apart from the aubergines in a pot of boiling water for a minute, allow them to cool and then add to the marinade mixture. Stir well and allow them to marinate overnight, if possible. Before cooking, soak some bamboo sticks in water for about an hour, then thread the vegetables on and roast the kebabs in an oven preheated to 200°C/gas mark 6 for about 30 minutes, turning frequently and basting them with the left-over marinade.

Hearty vegetable soup

2 celery sticks, chopped
2 medium-sized onions, chopped
1 large carrot, chopped
1 x 400g tin of chopped Italian tomatoes
700ml tomato juice
1 leek, chopped
1 Jerusalem artichoke (optional), chopped
1 sweet potato, chopped
1 x 400g tin of chickpeas, drained
1 x 400g tin of sweetcorn (with no salt or sugar added), drained
1 x 400g tin of butter beans (also drained)
150g brown basmati rice
2 teaspoons of soy sauce
2 teaspoons of thyme
1 teaspoon of ground black pepper
3 garlic cloves, crushed
2 tablespoons of dill

Combine all the ingredients in a large pot with 450ml of water and place over a high heat. Bring to the boil, then simmer for 30–40 minutes, until the vegetables are tender and the rice is cooked through.

Dinner

Roasted asparagus

1 bunch of asparagus
2 tablespoons of olive oil
juice of half a lemon
herbs (optional)
mustard powder (optional)

This is an easy one. You need at least one bunch of asparagus. Pre-heat the oven to 200°C/gas mark 6. Simply break off your asparagus where it bends naturally, rinse it and put it in an ovenproof dish. Cover it with the olive oil and lemon juice. Roast it in the oven for about 10 minutes; the spears should still be crisp. You can add all sorts of different herbs to your oil and lemon topping – such as dill or basil – or stir in a little mustard powder for some bite.

Roasted beetroot

5 or 6 baby beetroots
2 or 3 squeezes of lemon juice
3 garlic cloves, crushed
For the dressing:
2 tablespoons of olive oil
5 garlic cloves, minced
2 tablespoons of either organic balsamic vinegar, apple cider vinegar or lemon juice

Wash and trim the beetroots. Mix together the dressing ingredients. Preheat the oven to 200°C/gas mark 6, and place the beets in a baking tray with 120ml of water and the lemon juice. Add the garlic cloves to the water around the base of the beets. Roast for about 10 minutes, then drain off the liquid and pour over the dressing instead. Cook for another 5 minutes and then serve.

Butter bean mash

2 or 3 x 400g tins of butter beans
1 teaspoon of vegan stock powder
3 tablespoons of chopped fresh parsley
2 tablespoons of freshly cut chives
2 tablespoons of live yoghurt (or, if you are dairy-free, 2 tablespoons of unsweetened soya milk)
freshly ground pepper

Drain and rinse the beans and cook them until they are really tender. Place in a food processor or liquidiser and add the other ingredients. Blend, and check the taste; season with sea salt if you need more flavour.

Chickpea curry

1 tablespoon of olive oil
1 medium-sized onion, chopped
2 garlic cloves, crushed
5cm piece of root ginger, grated
$\frac{1}{4}$ teaspoon of chilli powder (mild)
$\frac{1}{2}$ teaspoon of ground cumin
$\frac{1}{4}$ teaspoon of ground coriander
$\frac{1}{4}$ teaspoon of turmeric
a pinch of sea salt
1 large tomato, chopped
a pinch of nitrate-free garam masala
2 x 400g tins of chickpeas, drained
To serve:
fresh ginger
garam masala

Put the olive oil, onion, garlic and ginger in a deep saucepan or wok. Cook until the onions are browned and slightly caramelised. Next, add the chilli powder, cumin, coriander, turmeric and sea salt. Allow the flavours to merge for a couple of minutes, and then add the chopped tomato along with the garam masala.

Cook until the sauce begins to thicken, then add 120ml of water and continue cooking. Tip in the chickpeas and stir everything together. Continue cooking, allowing the chickpeas to soften, and mash a few during the process. When you serve the curry, grate a little fresh ginger over the top and sprinkle with garam masala.

Creamy fish pie with pine nut crust

2 tablespoons of olive oil
1 leek, thinly sliced
2 carrots, very thinly sliced
1 teaspoon of freshly ground pepper
1 teaspoon of grated nutmeg
2 pinches of sea salt
1 fresh bay leaf
2 tablespoons of parsley
1 teaspoon of freshly cut chives
1 handful of fresh tarragon leaves
2 tablespoons of cornflour
125ml of natural live yoghurt *or* 125ml of unsweetened soya milk
1 medium fillet of pollack or haddock
1 medium fillet of naturally smoked haddock or mackerel
1 fillet of salmon
2 handfuls of mangetout
about 8 baby sweetcorn cobs
butter bean mash (see page 133) or sweet potato and parsnip mash (see page 139)
2 good handfuls of pine nuts

Preheat the oven to 180°C/gas mark 4. In a wok or a large saucepan, heat the olive oil and soften the leek and carrots. Add the pepper, nutmeg, sea salt, bay leaf, parsley, freshly cut chives and tarragon leaves. Whisk the cornflour into the live yoghurt or unsweetened soya milk, and add to the pan, stirring it in well.

Add the fillets of fish – roughly 400g in total. As they cook, gently break them into chunks. Throw in the mangetout and baby sweetcorn cobs. Stir as the mixture thickens and then decant it into an ovenproof container, removing the bay leaf. Top with butter bean mash (or sweet potato and parsnip mash) into which you have stirred the pine nuts, and place in the oven for 15 minutes until heated through.

Fish (or tofu) and lemon tagine with green olives

1 teaspoon of ground cumin
1 teaspoon of ground cinnamon
1 teaspoon of ground coriander
1 teaspoon of paprika
1 teaspoon of cayenne pepper
sea salt and freshly ground pepper
2 or 3 fillets (400g) of firm white fish such as haddock or pollack (or 2 large chunks of tofu)
olive oil
600ml low-sodium vegan vegetable stock
1 handful of finely chopped coriander
3 thinly sliced preserved lemons (plus a little of the brine)
1 handful of pitted green olives
zest of 1 lemon
To serve:
freshly cut coriander

Preheat the oven to 140°C/gas mark 1. You can use any firm white fish, chicken (when you are off the programme) or tofu for this dish. To begin with, blend the spices, salt and pepper. Cover the fish or tofu with the mixture and allow to settle for 10 minutes. Warm some olive oil in a large ovenproof pan which you can also put on the hob, and gently sauté the fish or tofu until browned on all sides. Next, add the vegetable stock, coriander, preserved lemons and brine and green olives. Bring to the boil, then cook in the oven for 90 minutes, stirring frequently.

Before serving, stir the lemon zest into the mixture; garnish with a good handful of freshly cut coriander.

Lentil moussaka

250g of lentils
2 small aubergines
4 sweet potatoes
5 tomatoes
2 courgettes
olive oil
1 x 400g tin of chopped tomatoes
2 carrots, chopped
1 fennel bulb, chopped
2 bay leaves
3 big handfuls of fresh spinach
1 teaspoon of cayenne pepper
2 teaspoons of oregano
2 teaspoons of basil
3 garlic cloves, crushed
2 medium-sized onions, very finely sliced
1 teaspoon of ground cinnamon
sea salt
black pepper
1 big carton (at least 500ml) of plain live yoghurt
1 egg
nutmeg
feta cheese (optional)

Begin by cooking the lentils according to the instructions on the packet. Slice the aubergines, sweet potatoes, tomatoes and courgettes. Brush with olive oil and place under the grill for about 7 minutes, turning halfway through. When your lentils are cooked, rinse them carefully, and add the tinned chopped tomatoes, carrots, fennel bulb, bay leaves, spinach, cayenne pepper, oregano, basil, garlic, onions, cinnamon, a little sea salt and some black pepper. Cook for 20 minutes, until all the chopped vegetables are soft.

Preheat the oven to 200°C/gas mark 6. Mix the carton of yoghurt with the egg, a grating of nutmeg and plenty of fresh pepper. Get a good-sized casserole dish, and layer your sliced vegetables. Start with a layer of sweet potatoes and aubergines, top with courgettes, and then ladle on the lentil mix, removing the bay leaves. Cover with about half of the creamy yoghurt mixture, and then repeat. Continue until you have used all the ingredients, reserving about 125ml of the yoghurt mixture till the end. Finish off with a lentil layer, and then cover with the yoghurt. If you are doing the 30-day plan, you can crumble feta cheese over top. Otherwise, we would suggest a good grating of nutmeg. Bake for 30 minutes, until bubbling.

Honey-roasted salmon

4 or 5 salmon fillets
2 tablespoons of honey (Manuka is best; see page 101)
1 tablespoon of lemon juice
2 tablespoons of fresh dill

This couldn't be easier, and it's a delicious way to enjoy one of the most nutritious fishes around. You need 4 or 5 salmon fillets for this quantity of topping, so you can either make extra or save your topping for another day.

Preheat the oven to 200°C/gas mark 6. Simply blend together the honey, lemon juice and dill and spread on top of the salmon pieces. Roast for about 10–15 minutes, until the topping is bubbling and the inside is nicely flushed rather than white or pink.

Sesame stir-fry

For the base sauce:
5cm of fresh ginger, grated
3 tablespoons of sesame oil
2 tablespoons of rice vinegar (or, if you prefer, the same quantity of grapefruit juice)
2 handfuls of chopped coriander
4 garlic cloves, minced
1 teaspoon of lime juice
sea salt
freshly ground pepper
For the stir-fry:
olive oil
sesame seeds
your choice of vegetables, such as sugar snap peas, mangetout, baby carrots, baby sweetcorn, chopped kale, Chinese cabbage, broccoli, cauliflower, courgettes or peppers
To serve:
steamed fish or tofu (optional)

This is an easy one. Choose any fish you like or some tofu, or simply go it alone with veggies – but keep the emphasis on the vegetables if you do decide to use fish or tofu. (Steam the fish or tofu if you do want to use them.) The important thing to remember is that root vegetables, such as parsnips, carrots, and sweet potatoes will take about 10 minutes longer than anything else. To make this work, it's easiest to test your veggies as you go. They should break when prodded with a fork but don't let them get too soggy. If any are ready before the rest, remove them on to a heated plate, and replace them later on.

Begin by making a base sauce: mix together all the ingredients and put to one side to let the flavours develop.

In a wok or a heavy-based saucepan, heat a little olive oil with a few sesame seeds or, if you don't have them, sesame oil. Drop in any combination of vegetables – anything goes! When they start to sizzle a little, pour in your sauce. Turn off the heat and let the vegetables absorb the flavours for about an hour or so. When you are ready to serve, quickly reheat and the flavour will be rich and beautiful. Serve with the steamed fish or tofu, if using, or you could drop your tofu into the blend when you add the sauce. Delicious!

Sweet potato and parsnip mash

2 large sweet potatoes
2 large parsnips
black pepper
sea salt
olive oil
plain live yoghurt, unsweetened soya milk or vegan stock

To retain as many nutrients as possible, it's best to bake the potatoes and parsnips in their skins, let them cool, and then peel them. In a large saucepan, mash the insides of the vegetables together with a good grating of black pepper, a pinch of sea salt, a teaspoon of olive oil and, if desired, a few tablespoons of plain live yoghurt. If you want to give dairy a miss, you can use a little unsweetened soya milk, or, better still, a little vegan stock. Heat gently until warmed through, stirring frequently to make sure it doesn't catch.

Stir-fried tofu with winter vegetables

a good selection of winter vegetables: parsnips, squash, turnip, sweet potatoes, Jerusalem artichoke, carrots and fennel
olive oil
3 garlic cloves
2 tablespoons of honey
1 tablespoon of sesame oil
1 red chilli, very finely chopped
a pinch of Chinese five spice powder
150g tofu

Winter vegetables are a delight, and can easily be incorporated into most dishes. Chop a variety of them into very thin strips. Blanch in boiling water for a few minutes, then refresh them in cold water. Heat a little olive oil in a wok, and crush the garlic into the oil. Heat for a moment, and then add the honey, sesame oil, chilli and Chinese five spice powder. Chop the tofu into good-sized squares and sauté these quickly until lightly browned. Add your vegetables, and stir-fry until heated through. Serve with rice.

Tuna skewers

1 tablespoon of freshly grated ginger
4 garlic cloves, crushed
¼ teaspoon of cayenne pepper
1 teaspoon of ground coriander
½ teaspoon of turmeric
1 teaspoon of sea salt
fresh black pepper
3 tablespoons of olive oil
2 or 3 good-quality tuna steaks

You'll need to get some good, chunky tuna steaks for this one; however, you don't need much; the flavouring is so satisfying that a little goes a long way. You can also use the same spices for other fish dishes, although they may be a little more difficult to thread …

Mix together the ginger, garlic, cayenne pepper, ground coriander, turmeric, sea salt, a good grating of fresh black pepper and the olive oil. Cut the tuna steaks into chunks. You don't have to use all the tuna in the kebabs; you can set one steak aside after marinating and use it in a Niçoise salad or for sandwiches at a later date. Rub the marinade into the steaks and refrigerate for at least an hour. Thread pieces of tuna on to a skewer and grill until the outsides are bubbling and the insides are still slightly pink.

Salads

Salads are easy and can make a tasty lunch or dinner. Anything goes with them; the idea is to include many fresh, raw or even cooked varieties of vegetables and fruit in your daily diet. Toss together some leftover veggies from the night before, a handful of chopped fresh fruit or nuts, some feta or goat's cheese if it's on your menu – and then pile it on to some delicious and nutritious greens of any description.

Three-bean salad

125g green beans, cut into halves
2 tablespoons of olive oil
2 tablespoons of lemon juice
1 teaspoon of smoked paprika
2 garlic cloves, crushed
1 x 400g tin of cannellini or red kidney beans, drained
1 x 400g tin of black-eyed beans, drained
6 spring onions
1 handful of finely chopped parsley
1 handful of finely chopped coriander
black pepper
feta cheese (optional)

Stir together the green beans, olive oil, lemon juice, smoked paprika, garlic, cannellini or red kidney beans, black-eyed beans and spring onions. Let them marinate together in the fridge for an hour or two, and then stir in the parsley and coriander. Serve with a good sprinkling of black pepper. If you are on the 30-day programme, why not add some chunks of feta cheese before serving?

Beetroot salad

10 baby beetroots, with leaves
150g of rocket
150g of sugar snap peas, blanched
2 peeled blood oranges, sectioned and sliced
3 tablespoons of olive oil
1½ tablespoons of lemon juice
2 teaspoons of chopped oregano (fresh, if possible; halve the amount, if not)
a pinch of sea salt
freshly ground pepper

Trim the baby beetroots, reserving some of the best of the smallest leaves. Cook the beets in boiling water for 30–40 minutes, until tender. Rinse under running water and peel away the skin. Next, arrange the beetroot leaves, rocket, blanched sugar snap peas (you can do this by dropping them in a pot of boiling water for 1 minute and then refreshing them in ice-cold water) and blood oranges. Then mix together the rest of the ingredients and pour over the salad.

Carrot salad

1kg of carrots
2 garlic cloves, crushed
4 tablespoons of lemon juice
4 tablespoons of virgin olive oil
2 teaspoons of sweet paprika
2 teaspoons of ground cumin
1 teaspoon of sea salt
freshly ground black pepper
2 good handfuls of fresh mint leaves
about 12 black olives, sliced
150g of feta cheese (optional)
sunflower seeds

Peel and slice the carrots and cook them in boiling water for 1 minute. Take them out and refresh them in a bowl of ice-cold water. Drain them well, and put them in a large bowl. Next, mix together the garlic, lemon juice, olive oil, sweet paprika, cumin, sea salt and lots of freshly ground black pepper. Pour this over the carrots, and cover them with the mint leaves, black olives and, if you are doing the 30-day programme, the feta cheese. If you aren't doing dairy, I would suggest letting the salad marinate for a while before serving, and then topping it with lightly warmed sunflower seeds.

Lentil salad with walnuts and goat's cheese

2 roundels of goat's cheese cut into 1cm slices
olive oil
2 x 400g tins of puy lentils, drained
2 tablespoons of walnut oil
2 tablespoons of sherry vinegar
200g of walnuts
at least 25g of fresh chives, finely chopped

This is one for the 30-day programme only; the lentil salad is, however, delicious without the cheese. Though this salad can be kept for later, you need to prepare the cheese just before you are ready to serve it. As it is, it serves two to three; if you're eating by yourself one roundel of cheese would be fine – save the rest of the salad for later.

Brush both sides of the goat's cheese with olive oil and set to one side. Mix together the puy lentils, walnut oil, sherry vinegar, walnuts and fresh chives. Put this mix in the fridge to the allow the flavours to blend while you cook the cheese. Place the goat's cheese on foil and grill until bubbling. Give each person a portion of the cool lentil salad and place the goat's cheese on top.

Warm, fruity quinoa salad

250g of fruity quinoa recipe (see page 126)
2 handfuls of coriander leaves
2 handfuls of fresh parsley
3 handfuls of wilted spinach
2 tablespoons of honey and lemon dressing (see page 145)

Cook the quinoa according to the recipe, omitting the yoghurt or rice milk. Cool after cooking, then add the coriander and parsley and place in the fridge. Serve at room temperature, topped with the spinach and the dressing, warmed to slightly bubbling.

Warm watercress salad

500g of fresh watercress
4 tablespoons of olive oil
½ teaspoon of sesame oil
½ teaspoon of flaxseed oil
2 tablespoons of organic balsamic vinegar
1 tablespoon of grapefruit juice
lots of freshly ground pepper

Wash and trim the watercress. Make the dressing by mixing the rest of the ingredients together. Heat the dressing over a low heat until just bubbling, and then set it to one side for the flavours to mature. When it is hand hot, pour it over the watercress and serve.

Why not also try:

- Apple, pear, walnut and goat's cheese on a bed of rocket.
- Blanched green beans, almonds, broccoli spears and red pepper strips on any bed of soft greens.
- Spinach with a hard-boiled egg, lightly toasted sunflower seeds and a little feta.

- Dried apricots, apple and walnuts on Romaine lettuce.
- Berries of any description with a variety of lightly toasted nuts, served on a bed of greens.
- Radishes, cucumber, spring onions, cherry tomatoes and edamame beans, doused in vinaigrette and gently tossed with summer leaves.
- Melon, poppy seeds and lettuce leaves with a fresh dressing (try the sweet orange dressing on page 146).
- Raw broccoli, chopped red onion, lightly toasted sunflower seeds, grapes, dried cranberries and raisins in a light honey vinaigrette.
- Freshly grated beetroot with a good handful of chopped coriander, the same of mint, the juice of a lemon, and all tossed together with some fresh live yoghurt.
- Cherry tomatoes with red onion, fresh spinach, watercress, fresh basil and a good clove or two of garlic, sprinkled with some balsamic vinegar and olive oil.
- Chickpeas with a lemon vinaigrette, plenty of chopped cucumber, chives and coriander, and a little bit of freshly chopped chilli pepper. If you like your chickpeas sweet, blend with mint, raisins, red onions and dried cranberries and use a honey and lemon dressing instead (see below).

Easy dressings, dips and sauces

Honey and lemon dressing

2 tablespoons of honey (Manuka is best, see page 101)
3 tablespoons of freshly squeezed lemon juice
3 tablespoons of olive oil
a pinch of sea salt
a good grind of black peppercorns
¼ teaspoon of mustard powder (optional)

Blend together all the ingredients. If you like a little more tang, use the mustard powder and shake before serving.

Lemon herb dressing

125ml freshly squeezed lemon juice
zest of 1 lemon
125ml olive oil
at least 2 or 3 fresh green herbs, such as chives, chervil, coriander, parsley, basil, thyme or dill – the more the better
1 garlic clove, crushed
honey
sea salt
black pepper

Anything goes with this recipe! Begin with a base of the lemon juice, lemon zest and olive oil. Then finely chop the green herbs, allow them to marinate in the oil and juice for about 24 hours in the fridge, then shake and add the garlic. Leave for another 12–24 hours, then strain out the herbs. Stir in a little honey, a pinch of sea salt and a good grinding of black pepper, and shake well before using.

Sweet orange dressing

2 teaspoons of honey
125ml of freshly squeezed orange juice
zest of 1 orange
1 teaspoon of lemon juice
120ml olive oil
a pinch of salt
a tiny pinch of dried tarragon

Blend all the ingredients and shake before serving.

Fresh oregano dressing

a good handful of fresh oregano leaves
2 pinches of sea salt
5 black peppercorns
1 teaspoon of mustard powder
1 garlic clove, finely chopped
3 tablespoons of lemon juice or red wine vinegar
3 tablespoons of olive oil
chilli powder

In a mortar and pestle, crush the oregano leaves with the sea salt, black peppercorns, mustard powder and garlic. When you have a good paste, shake it together in a jar – make sure the lid is firmly on – with the lemon juice or red wine vinegar, along with the olive oil and a small pinch or two of chilli powder, or as much as you like, but don't over-whelm the oregano. Shake well before serving.

Black bean hummus

1 x 400g tin of black beans, drained
6 tablespoons of roasted tahini
2 garlic cloves, minced
1 tablespoon of olive oil
1 teaspoon of lime juice
½ teaspoon of cumin

Blend all the ingredients in a liquidiser until smooth. If the mixture is too thick, add a few drops each of olive oil and lime juice.

Chickpea hummus

4 garlic cloves
2 x 400g tins of chickpeas, drained
175ml of roasted tahini

5 tablespoons of freshly squeezed lemon juice
125ml water
75ml olive oil
a pinch of sea salt
To garnish:
pine nuts
chopped fresh parsley

Blend all the hummus ingredients in a liquidiser until smooth. Top with pine nuts and parsley for a healthy garnish.

Crunchy guacamole

3 large, ripe avocados
3 spring onions, chopped
1 ripe tomato, chopped
1 small red chilli pepper, finely chopped
1 large bunch of coriander, chopped
1 good handful of mixed seeds (such as sunflower, sesame, flax, hemp and pumpkin)
2 garlic cloves, crushed
juice of 1 lemon

Mash the avocados and mix them together with the spring onions, tomato and red chilli pepper. Add the other ingredients. Serve immediately or store in an airtight container until required.

Honey and lemon dip

juice and zest of 1 lemon
2 tablespoons of honey

Simply add the lemon juice and zest to the honey, mix well and use as a sweet addition to fresh fruit crudités or to pour over fresh live yoghurt. Add to yoghurt with a grating of cinnamon for a delicious dessert.

Mango chilli veggie dip

6 tablespoons of puréed mango (use tinned, or purée a large raw mango in a blender or food processor)
1 red chilli without the seeds, finely chopped
1 great big handful of coriander
1 teaspoon of sea salt
a few tablespoons of chopped spring onion
250ml of plain live yoghurt

Whizz all the ingredients in the blender and serve. It will keep for 48 hours in the fridge, and can be used as a vegetable dip or as an accompaniment for fish or tofu.

Caramelised onion dip

2 or 3 medium onions, finely chopped
olive oil
1 garlic clove, crushed
fresh ginger
1 tablespoon of fresh chives
125ml fresh live yoghurt

Stir the onions gently in a little olive oil in a heavy-bottomed pan until browned and fragrant. Add the garlic and a grating of fresh ginger. Cook until lightly caramelised. Next, add the chives and take the pan off the heat. Transfer the onion mixture to a bowl and allow it to cool a little. Stir in the yoghurt and refrigerate for 2 hours to allow the flavours to blend. Serve with fresh crudités, oatcakes or as an accompaniment to any savoury dish.

Pea hummus

2 mugfuls of fresh peas
2 garlic cloves
juice of half a lemon
2 tablespoons of roasted tahini
a pinch of sea salt
a good grating of black pepper
1 tablespoon of cumin
1 tablespoon of olive oil

Blend all the ingredients in a liquidiser until smooth.

Spinach raita

350g of trimmed spinach
600g plain live yoghurt
3 garlic cloves, crushed
a pinch of sea salt
black pepper

Wash the spinach and place in a pan over medium heat with just the water clinging to its leaves. Cover and cook for 3–5 minutes until wilted, stirring occasionally. Drain and squeeze out the water. Add to the yoghurt, along with the garlic, sea salt and some black pepper to taste. Not only is this the perfect accompaniment for fish and tofu, but it can also be used with beef and chicken at a later date. It makes a lovely base for a rye bread open sandwich, served with some steamed salmon or a sliced hard-boiled egg.

Tzaziki

3 garlic cloves
2 good handfuls each of parsley, coriander and mint
½ a cucumber, finely chopped
1 small red chilli, very finely chopped
500g of plain live yoghurt
sea salt
black pepper

This is a delicious dip or accompaniment to fish, tofu or even vegetables. Blend the garlic with the parsley, coriander and mint. Stir in the cucumber and red chilli. Add the yoghurt and season with a little sea salt and black pepper. Stir well and let the flavours mingle for at least an hour before serving. This will sit for a day or two in the fridge, but stir it frequently.

Fresh fruit purée

No need for cooking here! Choose very ripe fruits such as raspberries, strawberries, papaya, mango or pears. Mash them and put the resulting mixture into a firm sieve; put the sieve over a bowl and push the fruit mash through the mesh into the bowl. Don't forget to scrape the underneath of the sieve into the bowl. Use this juice to flavour dishes, to top non-wheat toast or fresh, live yoghurt. If you want a little more bite to your purée, give the sieve a miss, and purée the lot in a liquidiser, with a touch of lemon juice to preserve it and a little honey to keep it sweet. If you like it thicker, sprinkle a little cornflour over the blend before you purée. You can heat this up for a variety of different recipes; however, in its raw form it provides the optimum number of nutrients. It will keep in the fridge for about 72 hours, covered.

Easy tomato sauce

3 garlic cloves
1 small onion
olive oil
1 handful of freshly chopped basil
several sprigs of finely chopped rosemary
1 bay leaf
1 tablespoon of honey
3 x 400g tins chopped plum tomatoes or 1kg fresh tomatoes, chopped
1 teaspoon of lemon juice
1 teaspoon of red wine vinegar
2 pinches of sea salt
coarsely ground black pepper

It's a good idea to keep a few pots of this in the freezer, as it makes an ideal last-minute pasta sauce, and is also a good base for lentil or vegetable casseroles and stews. You can use fresh or tinned tomatoes, organic when you can, or tomato passata will work too.

Sauté the garlic and onion in a heavy-bottomed pan with the olive oil until softened. Add the basil, rosemary, bay leaf, honey and chopped tomatoes. Add 175ml of water along with the lemon juice and red wine vinegar, sea salt and some black pepper, and bring to the boil. Simmer the sauce for 20–30 minutes. Liquidise it if you want a smooth sauce.

Watercress pesto

2 garlic cloves
1 pinch of sea salt
1 tablespoon of walnut oil
2 tablespoons of walnut pieces
1 large bunch of chopped watercress leaves
1 tablespoon of olive oil
1 teaspoon of mustard powder
1½ tablespoons of freshly squeezed lemon juice

To garnish:
goat's cheese or feta (optional)
1 good handful of chives

In a liquidiser, blend together all the ingredients until smooth. If you are eating dairy, sprinkle with goat's cheese or feta, and a good handful of chives.

Serve the pesto with non-wheat, gluten-free pasta (corn, quinoa or rice pasta), or toss it with cooled brown rice to make a salad. Alternatively, you could add chopped raw vegetables to this pesto to make a crunchy salad, and use a sprinkling of watercress leaves and chopped walnuts as a garnish.

Puddings

Apple and raisin crumble

4 cooking apples
2 tablespoons of cornflour
3 teaspoons of cinnamon
2 teaspoons of honey
2 handfuls of raisins
2 teaspoons of lemon juice
freshly grated zest of 1 orange
2 handfuls of rolled oats
2 drops of pure vanilla essence
1 tablespoon of olive oil

Preheat the oven to 160°C/gas mark 2–3. Peel, core and thinly slice the apples. Toss them with the cornflour, 1 teaspoon of the cinnamon, the honey and raisins. Moisten the apple mixture with the lemon juice and orange zest. Next, mix together the rolled oats, the remaining 2 teaspoons of cinnamon, vanilla essence and olive oil. Cover the apples and raisins with the crumble mixture, and bake for 30 minutes.

Baked figs

8 figs
2 tablespoons of honey
zest of 1 lemon
1 lime
1 orange
120ml of water or grape juice

Preheat the oven to 200°C/gas mark 6. Place as many figs as you like upright – this works well with 8 – in an ovenproof dish with the other ingredients. Bake for about 20 minutes and serve.

Poached pears

2 or 3 conference pears, peeled
6 tablespoons of honey
2 large pieces of thinly pared lemon rind
juice of ½ a lemon
a few allspice berries
2 star anise
1 cinnamon stick
350ml of white grape juice
350ml of orange juice

Peel the pears, and set them to one side. If you need to make more, there'll be plenty of liquid to make it work, so go ahead and prepare some more. Preheat the oven to 180°C/gas mark 4. Put the rest of the ingredients in an ovenproof dish which you can also use on the hob and stir until they are combined. Now place the pears upright in the dish and make sure they are covered with liquid, adding a little more grape juice if necessary. Place on the hob and heat until the liquid begins to bubble, and then transfer to the oven for about another 20 minutes. Alternatively, you can continue to simmer them on the hob, covered, for the same length of time.

Peach and rhubarb compote

4 ripe peaches, peeled and sliced
4 or 5 good sticks of rhubarb, trimmed and chopped finely
250ml of freshly squeezed orange juice
1 cinnamon stick
a drop of vanilla essence
3 tablespoons of maple syrup

Place all the ingredients in a large saucepan. Bring to the boil and simmer until the fruit is soft and pliable. Remove from the heat and mash everything together, adding more orange juice or water as necessary. Serve hot or cold.

Pomegranate ice

1 large pomegranate
6 ice cubes
1 teaspoon of orange flower water
honey

Squeeze a large pomegranate over a bowl to catch the juice and loosen the seeds. Bang the skin with the back of a spoon or rolling pin to encourage the seeds to fall down into the bowl, and use a fork to pull out any that haven't succumbed to the pressure. Remove any pith from the bowl. Next, put the ice cubes and 1 tablespoon of water into a liquidiser and crush until the ice is in fine pieces; decant it into a serving bowl. Now scatter your pomegranate seeds and juice over the top, and sprinkle with a teaspoon of orange flower water blended with a little honey.

Fresh fruit and vegetable juices

Although fresh fruit and vegetable juices do not contain fibre, which is essential for the *Perfect Detox* programme, they are bursting with nutrients that will give your body the perfect boost. Sip on them throughout the day, or drink them with meals. If you suffer from blood-sugar problems, it might be a good idea to have a few nuts alongside, to prevent your glucose levels from soaring.

You'll need a good juicer for these, although if you are feeling inventive, you can most definitely use a food processor to mix the ingredients and then strain them through a fine sieve or a muslin cloth. If you find them a bit tart, add a little honey or maple syrup to sweeten, but not too much; you want to become used to the natural sweetness of foods while you detox. For all recipes, simply blend the ingredients together.

Apple celery

2 cored but unpeeled sweet apples
2 sticks of celery
¼ lemon

Bright beetroot

1 fresh beetroot, peeled
2 sticks of celery
150ml of red grape juice
1 carrot
2 kale leaves

Cherry grape

2 handfuls of fresh cherries, pitted
1 handful of red and green grapes, with seeds
1 lemon wedge, with the peel removed

Cucumber and apple

1 whole cucumber, unpeeled
1 apple, cored but unpeeled
2 sticks of celery
1 lemon wedge
5 mint leaves

Fragrant papaya

1 peeled papaya, with the seeds removed
1cm fresh ginger, peeled and sliced
1 lime wedge

Veggie cleanser

1 red pepper, chopped and deseeded
2 garlic cloves
any variety of greens, such as kale, spinach, watercress, lettuce, broccoli
or even organic carrot tops
1 fresh tomato
2 sticks of celery

Not sure what else goes well together? Why not test these out:
• Kiwi with celery and watercress.
• Apple with fresh green grapes, pear and celery.
• Carrot, ginger, tangerine and lemon.
• Spinach, lime and mango (not a pretty colour but very, very good
    for you).
• Blueberries, cranberries, cucumber and apple.
• Peach, apricot and carrot.
• Apple, red pepper, celery and cinnamon.

Conclusion

You now have all the tools you need to make informed choices about your diet and lifestyle. Even if you don't wish to undertake a long-term detoxification programme or, indeed, make any drastic changes to your diet, you can choose to eat or include foods and supplements that will support your overall health and encourage natural detoxification. Everything you do to assist your liver, and every other detox organ in your body, will encourage good health, and making small changes to what you eat or drink, and to the way you eat, can have a dramatic effect on how you look and feel.

There is no 'diet' that will cure the ills that are the result of a Western lifestyle; however, there are many, many things you can do to offset the damage. Whenever you can, take the opportunity to have a good clear-out, and in between, use the knowledge you've gained to make sensible choices towards good health. Most importantly, however, take note of everything around you and actively seek alternatives to the everyday options in our toxic world. Not only will you experience better health as a result, but you'll become a part of a new mindset and movement that may well prevent problems in the future.

So go on, let it all out!

Index

'acid-forming foods' 23
alcohol 20
aromatherapy oils 68–9
artichoke extract 63
artificial additives 20
ashwaganda 63

B-complex vitamins 59
baths, detoxification 69
beta-carotene 59, 75
biotin 59
breakfast 51–2
  recipes 124–6
breathing 35
buchu 64

caffeine 20–1
chelation therapy 78
choline 59
cleavers 64
coffee 20–1
  enemas 77–8
colon 13–14
colonic irrigation 77
cooking methods 49
cupping 78–9

dairy products 21–2
dandelion root 64
detox foot patches 76

detox plan
  14-day detox 32–41
  24-hour detox 28–32
  30-day detox 41–2
  adapting the
    programmes 42–3
  falling off the wagon 44
  side-effects of
    detoxing 43–6
detox therapies 76–81
detoxification baths 69
detoxing
  foods to avoid 19–27
  getting started 27
  other detox organs 13–15
  preparing for a detox
    17–19
  the role of your liver
    10–13
  toxic overload 8–10
  what does it involve? 16
  why detox? 15–16
'diet' foods 22
digestive enzymes 59–60
dinner 53–5
  recipes 132–40
dips 148–9
dressings 145–7
dry skin brushing 73

eggs 27

essential fatty acids (EFAs)
  61–2, 75
essential oils 68–9
exercise 34–6, 38

falling off the wagon 44
fasting 30
fatty foods 22–3
flower essences 70
folic acid 58
food preparation
  breakfast 51–2
  dinner 53–5
  lunch 52–3
  portion size 48
  puddings 55
  raw or cooked? 49
  snacks 55–6
  stuck for inspiration?
    56
  variety 48–9
  which cooking method?
    49
foods to avoid 19–26
foot patches, detox 76
fruit juices, fresh
  156–7
fruit purée, fresh 151

glutathione 61
guacamole 148

herbal remedies 62–7
Herxheimer Reaction 43–4
homeopathic remedies 70–2
hummus 147, 150

juniper berries 65

kidneys 13

lifestyle 34–9
liver
  role of your 10–11
  symptoms of an over-worked or toxic liver 11–13
'low-cal' foods 22
lunch 52–3
  recipes 127–31
lungs 14
lymphatic system 14–15

magnesium 58
manual lymphatic drainage 77
massage 76–7
measures 123
meat 23
meditation 80–1
milk thistle 65
molybdenum 59
MSM 75
mucoid plaque 23
multivitamins and minerals 57–9

natural skincare products 73–4

organic foods 50–1

pesto 152–3
Pine Bark Extract 75
portions 48, 123
potassium 58
potatoes 24
poultry 23
prebiotics 61
probiotics 61
psyllium husks and seeds 66
puddings 55, 153–5

raita 150
raw/cooked food 49
ready meals 24–5
red clover 66
refined carbohydrates 25–6
relaxation 38, 79–81

salads 141–5
salt 25
SAMe 60
sauces 24–5
saunas 72
schizandra 66
selenium 59
side-effects 43–6
skin 14
  care of 36–8

clean 73
detoxification 72–5
dry skin brushing 73
nourishing 74–5
sleep 38–9
slippery elm 67
snacks 55–6
steam rooms 72
steaming food 49
stir-fries 49
sugar 25–6
supplements 57–62

tea 21
tomato sauce 152
toxic overload 8–10
toxins 8
tzaziki 151

uva ursi 67

varied diet 48–9
vegetable juices, fresh 156–7
vitamins, B-complex 59

wheat 26
wheatgrass 26
whole-body relaxation 79–80

yarrow 67

zinc 58